Life Under CONTROL

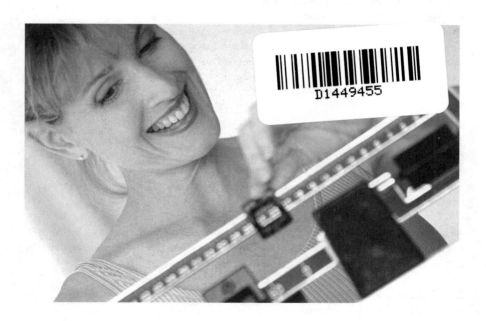

Gospel Light

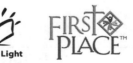
FIRST PLACE™

Gospel Light is an evangelical Christian publisher dedicated to serving the local church. We believe God's vision for Gospel Light is to provide church leaders with biblical, user-friendly materials that will help them evangelize, disciple and minister to children, youth and families.

It is our prayer that this Gospel Light resource will help you discover biblical truth for your own life and help you minister to others. May God richly bless you.

For a free catalog of resources from Gospel Light, please contact your Christian supplier or contact us at 1-800-4-GOSPEL or www.gospellight.com.

PUBLISHING STAFF
William T. Greig, Chairman
Kyle Duncan, Publisher
Dr. Elmer L. Towns, Senior Consulting Publisher
Pam Weston, Senior Editor
Patti Pennington Virtue, Associate Editor
Jeff Kempton, Editorial Assistant
Hilary Young, Editorial Assistant
Bayard Taylor, M.Div., Senior Editor, Biblical and Theological Issues
Barbara LeVan Fisher, Packaging Concept and Design
Samantha A. Hsu, Cover and Internal Designer

CAUTION

The information contained in this book is intended to be solely informational and educational. It is assumed that the First Place participant will consult a medical or health professional before beginning this or any other weight-loss or physical fitness program.

CONTENTS

FOREWORD

My introduction to Bible study came when I joined First Place in March of 1981. I had been in church since I was a small child, but the extent of my study of the Bible had been reading my Sunday School quarterly on Saturday night. On Sunday morning, I would listen to my Sunday School teacher as she taught God's Word to me. During the worship service, I would listen to our pastor as he taught God's Word to me. Digging out the truths of the Bible for myself had frankly never entered my mind.

Perhaps you are right where I was back in 1981. If so, you are in for a blessing you never dreamed possible. As you start studying the truths of the Bible for yourself, you will see God begin to open your understanding of His Word. Bible study is one of the nine commitments of the First Place program. The First Place Bible studies are designed to be done on a daily basis. Each day's study will take approximately 15 to 20 minutes to complete, but you will be discovering the deep truths of God's Word as you work through each week's study.

There are many in-depth Bible studies on the market. The First Place Bible studies are not designed for the purpose of in-depth study. They are designed to be used in conjunction with the other eight commitments of the program to bring balance into our lives. Our desire is for each member to begin having a personal quiet time with God each day. This time alone with God should include a time of prayer, Bible reading and Bible study. Having a quiet time is a daily discipline that will bring the rich rewards of balance, something we all need.

A part of each week's study is the Bible memory verse for the week. You will find a CD at the back of this Bible study that contains all 10 of the memory verses for the study set to music. The CD has an upbeat tempo suitable for use when exercising. The songs help you to easily memorize the verses and retain them for future reference. If you memorize Scripture as you study, God will use His Word to transform your life.

Almost every First Place member I have talked with about the program says, "The weight loss is wonderful, but the most important thing I have received from my association with First Place is learning to study God's Word."

God bless you as you begin this exciting journey toward a balanced life. God will richly bless your efforts to give Him first place in your life. Remember Matthew 6:33: "But seek first his kingdom and his righteousness, and all these things will be given to you as well."

Carole Lewis
First Place National Director

INTRODUCTION

The First Place Bible studies were developed to be used in conjunction with the First Place weight-loss program. However, the studies could also be used by anyone who desires to learn more about God's Word and His will, with the added bonus of learning more about living a healthy lifestyle.

A Balanced Life

First Place is a Christ-centered health program, emphasizing balance in the physical, mental, emotional and spiritual areas of life. The First Place program is meant to be a daily process. As we learn to keep Christ first in our lives, we will find that He is the One who satisfies our hunger and our every need.

God's Word contains guidelines for maintaining our physical well-being, equipping us mentally to make right choices, providing emotional stability to handle everyday circumstances as well as crisis situation, and growing spiritually as we deepen our relationship with Him.

The Nine Commitments

The First Place program has nine commitments that will help you draw closer to the Lord and aid you in establishing a solid, consistent and healthy Christian life. Each commitment is a necessary and important part of the goal of First Place: to help you become healthier and stronger in all areas of your life and live the abundant life He has planned for you. To help you achieve growth in all four areas, First Place asks you to keep these nine commitments:

1. Attendance
2. Encouragement
3. Prayer
4. Bible Reading
5. Scripture Memory Verse
6. Bible Study
7. Live-It Plan
8. Commitment Record
9. Exercise

The Components

There are six distinct components to this Bible study to aid you in bringing balance to your life. These components include the 10-week Bible study, 6 Wellness Worksheets, 2 weeks of menu plans, the leader's discussion guide, 13 Commitment Records and the Scripture memory CD.

The Bible Study

Each week of each 10-week Bible study is divided into five daily assignments with days 6 and 7 set aside for reflections on the week's lesson. The following guidelines will help make your study more enjoyable and profitable:

- Set aside 15 to 20 minutes each day to complete the daily assignment. It's best not to attempt to complete a week's worth of Bible study in one day.
- Pray before each day's study and ask God to give you understanding and a teachable heart.
- Keep in mind that the ultimate goal of Bible study is not for knowledge only but also for application and a changed life.
- First Place suggests using the *New International Version* of the Bible to complete the studies.
- Don't feel anxious if you can't seem to find the *correct* answer. Many times the Word will speak differently to different people, depending upon where they are in their walk with God and the season of life they are experiencing.
- Be prepared to discuss with your fellow First Place members what you learned that week through your study.

Wellness Worksheets

The informative and interactive Wellness Worksheets have been developed by Dr. Jody Wilkinson of the Cooper Institute in Dallas, Texas. These worksheets are intended to help you understand and achieve balance in all four areas of your life: physical, mental, emotional and spiritual. Your leader will assign specific worksheets as At-Home Assignments throughout the 13-week session.

Menu Plans

The two-week menu plans were developed especially for First Place by Chef Scott Wilson. Each menu is meant to simplify meal planning and include food exchanges. These meals are based on the MasterCook software that uses a database of over 6,000 food items, which was prepared using United States Department of Agriculture (USDA) publications and information from food manufacturers.

Leader's Discussion Guide

This discussion guide is provided to help the First Place leader guide a group through this Bible study. It provides information for the leader to prepare for each weekly group meeting.

Personal Weight Record

The Personal Weight Record is for the member to use to keep a record of weight loss. After the weigh-in at each week's meeting, the member will record any loss or gain on the chart.

Commitment Records

Thirteen Commitment Records (CRs) are provided in the back of this Bible study. For your convenience these have been printed on perforated paper so that you may easily remove them from the book and carry them with you through each week as you keep your First Place commitments. Directions for filling out the CRs precedes those pages.

Scripture Memory CD

Since Scripture memory is such a vital part of the First Place program, the Scripture memory CD for this study is included in the back inside cover. The verses for this study are set to music that can be listened to as you work, play or travel. The CD can be an effective tool as you exercise since the first verse is set to music with a warm-up tempo, the next eight verses are set to workout tempo, and the music of the last verse can be used for a cooldown.

LIFE OUT OF CONTROL

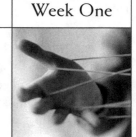

MEMORY VERSE

Restore to me the joy of your salvation
and grant me a willing spirit, to sustain me.
Psalm 51:12

Do you ever feel your life is out of control? If so, you have company—not only the people in your First Place group, but even a great spiritual leader in the Bible. You'll learn about him in your study this week.

Are you ready to get your life under control? Great! The studies you'll complete over the next 10 weeks will help you get your life under control—God's control. God's plan for your life includes His supernatural control in every part of your life: your thoughts, emotions, actions, tongue, relationships—everything in your life, including your health habits! Let's begin by learning why life slips out of control.

DAY 1: *A Life-Control Problem*

We all share a common problem. In our fast-paced culture, life can slip out of control. It happens to the best of us, including committed Christians. Life even slipped out of control for Israel's king, David, the one whom God referred to as "a man after his own heart" (1 Samuel 13:14). Read 1 Samuel 13:13-14 and Acts 13:22 and then answer the following:

➤ Why was God displeased with Saul?

≫ Why was God pleased with David?

King Saul had not kept God's commands, but God could say of David, "He will do everything I want him to do" (Acts 13:22). As a result, the nation of Israel thrived under David's leadership. David excelled in every area: military, political and spiritual. The tragedy, however, is that David hurt many with the sin in his later life.

As you read about David in 2 Samuel, write each step David took toward sin.

≫ 2 Samuel 11:2

≫ 2 Samuel 11:3

≫ 2 Samuel 11:4-5

≫ 2 Samuel 11:6-13

≫ 2 Samuel 11:14-15

For years David had served God faithfully, often in the most difficult of circumstances. In a matter of weeks, David's life spun out of control. The man after God's own heart crashed. Within a few weeks he had committed adultery with Bathsheba and then arranged the murder of her husband to cover up his sin.

➤ Does it surprise you that Paul still referred to David as a "man after [God's] own heart" (Acts 13:22) even though he was aware of David's failure? Why or why not?

Because of God's grace, He doesn't reject you when you fail. God continues to view you in light of your potential in Christ, not in the harsh light of current failure. God looks for your willingness to let go of the sin in true repentance. Later in this week's study you will learn how David came to grips with his sin when confronted with it.

When you are in Christ, your life can be under control—God's control. Fortunately, past problems, current struggles and temporary setbacks do not hinder God's ongoing work in your life. As He did with David, God offers you hope for getting life under control even after a crash.

➤ If God were to refer to you with a phrase that describes His assessment of your life in relation to Him, what phrase do you think He would use?

➤ According to Romans 8:6-8, what is the difference between the mind of a sinful man and the mind controlled by the Spirit?

➤ Read Romans 8:9-11. What promise is found in Romans 8:11?

God wants you to live as a person after His own heart. He sent the Holy Spirit to live in you and help you control your sinful nature. Be obedient and follow His will because He understands your struggles and weaknesses. You begin a new chapter each day, and the best part of the story can begin today.

Heavenly Father, I ask You today to help me live as the person You would have me to be. Open my ears and my eyes so that I may see and hear what You would have me do.

Father, give me a Spirit-controlled life so that I may be obedient and willing to do Your will in my life.

DAY 2: *Wrong Place at the Wrong Time*

David's story offers you good news: God forgives and rebuilds lives. However, God does not remove the consequences of uncontrolled actions. He didn't remove them for David; He won't remove them for you. Our challenge, then, is to learn from David's tragedy, so we can work to keep our lives under control. Even though David's sin involved adultery and murder, principles emerge from his experience that can be applied to our everyday lives. And you can use these spiritual principles to insure that your life stays under God's control.

The first principle learned from David's tragedy is that life can spin out of control when you are in the wrong place at the wrong time.

➤ According to 2 Samuel 11:1, where was David supposed to be?

➤ As you reread the story in 2 Samuel 11:1-14, list the things that would not have happened if David had been with his army.

We don't know why David wasn't fighting with his men. He may have had good reasons for staying behind in Jerusalem. Whatever the reasons, David's decision ultimately cost Uriah his life and set into motion negative repercussions within David's family and his nation. David made the choice to stay home—the wrong choice!

Psalm 25 focuses on the ways of the Lord. When you seek God's way and follow it, you limit the chances that you will be in the wrong place. Following His paths will lead you away from temptation and sin. Read the following verses from Psalm 25; then fill in the missing words of the following statements:

➤ Psalm 25:4   "Show me your ways, O LORD, teach me your
_____."

➤ Psalm 25:8   "He instructs _____ in his ways."

➤ Psalm 25:9   "He guides the _____ in what is right and teaches them his way."

➤ Psalm 25:10   "All the ways of the LORD are _____ and _____."

➤ When you are in the wrong place at the wrong time, what impact can it have on the areas in your life which are most tempting (such as overeating, lying, neglecting Bible study and prayer time and not exercising)?

When you seek God, He will show you His plans and way for your life so that you can follow Him and avoid sin.

Lord Jesus, thank You for loving me and teaching me Your ways so that I may stand before You without guilt.

Heavenly Father, I praise Your name because You made it possible for the Holy Spirit to live in me and guide me in the way that is right.

DAY 3: *The Dangerous Second Look*

Life can spin out of control when you begin to toy with sin. Like a rattlesnake on a road, sin is something from which we should flee. Both rattlesnakes and sin become more dangerous the closer you get or the longer you look!

➤ According to 2 Samuel 11:2-3, did David sin when he saw the woman bathing?

➤ How did David know she was beautiful?

➤ What did David do next?

With the first look, David might have said, "My, there's a woman bathing." The second look got him into trouble and enabled him to say, "My, that woman is beautiful." From that point on, David set his heart on a course doomed for destruction. With the second look, David began toying with sin and refused to stop. The second look caused him to act on what he saw and his life spun out of control.

James 1:14 describes what happens when things tempt you.

➤ When you take that second look at something that you know you should avoid, what things entice you?

➤ What practical advice is given in Proverbs 4:25-27?

If you toy with sin, your evil desires often overpower you. Even though you plan to take only a look, you often end up doing much more. This principle holds true in many areas of life, from sexual sin to overeating to unhealthy lifestyles.

➤ Second Corinthians 4:18 gives important advice about where to look to avoid sin. Write this verse in your own words.

So many times in your daily life you come across things that tempt you to take a second look. Many television shows, magazines and books portray situations that are undesirable and sinful. You can let your carnal nature be in control, or you can let the Holy Spirit be in control. The choice is yours to make. David made the wrong choice and paid for it dearly because sin has its consequences.

Father God, help me to keep my eyes so focused on Jesus that I will not be tempted to take a second look at sin.

Lord, show me Your way for my life, so I can follow You and avoid sin.

DAY 4: *Failure to Count the Cost of Sin*

Life can spin out of control when you think you can sin without consequences. Read 2 Samuel 11:4. The Bible affirms the beauty of Bathsheba. Nothing in the text suggests that David's night with her was not pleasurable. In the same way, sin is usually outwardly appealing and initially enjoyable.

➤ Do you agree or disagree with this observation of sin being outwardly appealing and enjoyable? Why?

➤ Have you seen this same principle at work in situations where you have been tempted with something so attractive and inviting that you overlooked the harm that may come from it? How?

Sin can be appealing and pleasurable—at least initially. However, another characteristic of sin counteracts the first two features. Sin always has consequences. David thought he could sin for a night without paying a price. The Bible is clear: sin brings inevitable consequences.

How readily we can identify with Paul! Like him, we can say, "I do not understand what I do. For what I want to do I do not do, but what I hate I do" (Romans 7:15). This creates real frustration.

➤ What did Paul say in Romans 7:18 about his struggle with sin?

➤ What does Proverbs 6:27-29 say about the far-reaching effects of sin?

➤ According to Galatians 6:7, what are the consequences of sin?

➣ What were the consequences of David's sin in 2 Samuel 11:5?

➣ What realization does David express in Psalm 51:4?

David knew his sin was against God. No matter how other people respond to us and our sinful behavior, our ultimate challenge is in dealing with God. How incredible that God responds with love, forgiveness and grace!

➣ According to 1 John 1:9, what must we do to receive forgiveness for our sins?

Lord God, thank You that through Jesus Christ I can live in victory over sin.

Father, I pray that I will never believe the lies of Satan that sin doesn't have a price tag.

DAY 5: *Problems Hidden from Other People*

Life can spin out of control when you attempt to cover up your problems. It's easy to believe that if others know your failure and struggle, they will hurt rather than help you. Read 2 Samuel 11:6-27 to see how David tried to cover his sin.

➣ How did David try to cover his sin?

>> What was the result of his cover-up?

David sinned when he committed adultery with Bathsheba. That one sin created several serious consequences. As David tried to hide his sin, he compounded the problems, which escalated the consequences. Before the cycle of sin and cover-up was complete, David had multiplied his problems to a crushing level. The more David worked to hide his sin, the more his life spun out of control.

You may fear the responses of people to your problems, weaknesses or sin. Your concern, however, should focus on God's evaluation. Ultimately, you must deal with Him. Psalm 32:3-4 tells how David's cover-up affected him.

>> How did David's sin affect him?

>> Can you identify with him? How?

Spiritual cover-ups become a heavy load God doesn't want you to carry. God is not shocked by your sin and weakness. Whether the sin is as evil as adultery and murder, or as simple as overindulgence, the situation is compounded when you do not confront it head-on.

>> What do you think would have happened if David had confessed his sin to the people, made restitution to Uriah and used the opportunity to affirm God's law?

When Nathan finally confronted David with his sin, the prophet used a story about another man before David could see his own sin. Read the story in 2 Samuel 12:1-14.

➻ Why did Nathan have to use such a story for David?

➻ What was David's response to the story (see vv. 5-6)?

➻ What was David's response when told that he was the man (v. 13)?

➻ In Psalm 32:1-2,5, how did David describe God's response to his confession?

From the story of David, you learn that godly people experience times when life spins out of control. The good news you learn from David is that God offers forgiveness and control in life. No matter how bad things get, God can bring your life under control once again.

Heavenly Father, help me to face my problems head-on, no matter what people think and whether or not they help me.

Christ Jesus, thank You for bringing my life under control. Help me to learn how to live under Your control, so I might avoid future problems.

The nine commitments of First Place include Bible study, reading Scripture and memorizing Scripture. Exercise, healthy eating and drinking water will benefit your physical well-being, but studying God's Word and committing it to memory will strengthen and nourish your spiritual well-being. God is much more interested in what is going on in your spiritual life than in your physical life. This isn't to say that He doesn't care about your physical health. He's concerned about every area of your life. He wants your life to be under His control. If that is the case, He will help you with all areas of your life.

Your physical needs can become a stronghold in your life. Concern about a thinner body, better muscle tone or better appearance sometimes gets in the way of what God really wants for you. In her book *Praying God's Word*, Beth Moore defines a stronghold as "any argument or pretension that 'sets itself up against the knowledge of God.' . . . A stronghold is anything that exalts itself in our minds, 'pretending' to be bigger or more powerful than our God."[1] It doesn't matter what the stronghold is. If it steals your focus and causes you to feel overpowered, your Christian life can become ineffective—which is precisely the goal of Satan.

Beth Moore devotes a chapter to just about every stronghold or worldly sin that can come into your life. The key to overcoming strongholds is memorizing Scripture to use in time of temptation or when a stronghold threatens to undermine your determination to avoid it.

Prayer using Scripture as its focus will help to keep you on course. The following prayers reflect three scriptural verses that address the stronghold of idolatry. When a stronghold becomes a powerful force in your life, it is in danger of becoming an idol. These prayers using Scripture will help you to turn everything over to God.

My Father, You are the Lord my God. I desire to love You, listen to Your voice and hold fast to You, for You, Lord, are my life (see Deuteronomy 30:20).[2]

Oh, Lord, help me to lift my eyes and look to the heavens and acknowledge who created all these. You bring out the starry host one by one and call each of them by name. Because of Your great power and mighty strength, not one of them is missing (see Isaiah 40:26).[3]

For me, there is but one God, the Father, from whom all things came and for whom I live; and there is but one Lord, Jesus Christ, through whom all things came and through whom we live (see 1 Corinthians 8:6).[4]

DAY 7: *Reflections*

As you focus this week on getting your life under control, you may be asking how you can memorize so much Scripture week after week. When you fill your mind with God's Word, you are renewing your mind. His Word guards you against becoming a victim of your worst enemy, Satan.

From the life of David, you learn that godly people experience times when life spins out of control. Many factors influence this loss of control: being in the wrong place, toying with sin, miscalculating the consequences of sin and attempting to hide sin from others and from God. The good news we learn from David's story is that God offers forgiveness and control in life.

Many psalms written by David are prayers of confession; others are praise and adoration; others are supplications to God to take care of His people. Psalm 23 is one of the most memorized of the psalms. Short psalms such as this are easy to memorize. Personalize the Scripture by putting your name in it. Write the verses in your own words and apply them to your own life.

One way to memorize is to review the verse daily by reading it several times during the day. Eventually the words will settle in. Look at how David prayed in Psalm 51. He knew he had sinned against God and confessed it before God. Your body is God's temple, and when you abuse it with poor health habits, your sin against your own body is a sin against God. Pray for God's guidance in your life as you follow the nine commitments made to First Place. You may not be able to keep every one of them every day or every week, but God is faithful. Do your best, and let God take care of the rest.

Each week the reflection days will end with examples of Scripture prayers to help you get started with memorizing Scripture. Also, look for meaningful Scriptures as you read the Bible, and write them as prayers in your prayer journal. Each week's memory verse is a good place to start.

Father God, let the words of my mouth and the meditation of my heart be pleasing in Your sight, O Lord, my Rock and my Redeemer (see Psalm 19:14).

My Father, You have said that if my earthly house, this tent I live in, is destroyed, I have a building from You, O God: a house not made by human hands but an eternal home in the heavens (see 2 Corinthians 5:1).

My faithful Father, Your Word tells me to cast my cares on You, and You will sustain me and You will never let the righteous fall (see Psalm 55:22).

Father God, restore to me the joy of Your salvation and grant me a willing spirit, to sustain me (see Psalm 51:12).

Notes
1. Beth Moore, *Praying God's Word* (Nashville, TN: Broadman and Holman Publishers, 2000), p. 3.
2. Ibid., p. 22.
3. Ibid., p. 25.
4. Ibid., p. 26.

GROUP PRAYER REQUESTS   TODAY'S DATE:_____

NAME	REQUEST	RESULTS

LIFE UNDER CHRIST'S CONTROL

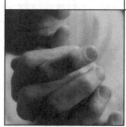

MEMORY VERSE

*May the God of hope fill you with all joy
and peace as you trust in Him, so that you may
overflow with hope by the power of the Holy Spirit.*

Romans 15:13

God has placed within you a human spirit which gives you the capacity for God's Holy Spirit to live in you and influence your thoughts, emotions and decisions. God never intended for you to attempt to keep life under control without His power. His presence in your life is essential for successful living.

In this week's study, you'll learn more about God's Holy Spirit. You'll discover the resources you have available through the Holy Spirit and the steps you can take to open your life fully to His work in you.

DAY 1: *Transformed by God's Holy Spirit*

Cars need gas. Lamps need electricity. You need God's Holy Spirit. When God designed your life, He planned to be actively involved with your daily life. Through His Spirit within you, God planned to provide all you need to live a life of positive, spiritual control.

➤ What analogy does 1 Corinthians 3:16 use to describe the believer's life?

➤ How do you feel about that analogy?

Throughout the Old Testament you will find references to the physical temple where the priests made sacrifices for the people. They entered the Holy of Holies to be in the presence of the Lord.

➤ In Habakkuk 2:20, what did the prophet say about the Temple?

The focus of the Old Testament was on the actual Temple building, a place of physical and spiritual beauty, as where God's presence was. In the New Testament, the focus shifted. The apostle Paul wrote that as a Christian, your body has become a temple of the Holy Spirit. That means that God's presence is with you; He is *in* you!

➤ What does 1 Corinthians 6:19-20 tell you about your body?

➤ In what ways do your actions indicate that God owns your life and your physical body? In what ways do your actions *not* indicate that God owns your life and your body?

God paid for your life through Christ's death on the cross. He owns you. Yet He entrusts your life and body to you so that you can glorify Him as you live. God is not, however, an absentee owner. He purchased your life, and then He took up residence within you through His Holy Spirit when you became a Christian.

➤ According to Ephesians 2:18, how do we as Christians have access to God?

Without Christ's death to pay for our sin, we would have remained God's enemy. Separated spiritually from God, we never could have enjoyed fellowship with God. Yet Christ's death and resurrection changed the situation. Now sin's price has been paid, and intimacy with God has become possible.

> According to 1 John 3:24, what is the evidence that shows you are a Christian?

The presence of God's Spirit in your life confirms that you have begun eternal life. Spiritual independence ends when we invite Christ to be Lord of our lives. Spiritual intimacy with God begins as God's Spirit enters our lives to control and empower us.

Thank You, Father God, for the relationship You made possible through the Holy Spirit in my life.

Lord God, I praise Your name for sending the Holy Spirit to live in me and empower me to keep my life under Your control.

DAY 2: *Filled with God's Spirit*

Not only has God designed your life so that He can live in you, but He also desires to be actively involved in your daily life. Through His Holy Spirit living in you, God wants to direct and empower you. Every aspect of your life is to be brought under His influence.

> What command does God give in Ephesians 5:18b?

≫ To what negative act does this verse contrast God's positive command?

When people are drunk with wine, it's clear that some outside force is influencing their behavior in a negative way. By contrast, God wants to have so much influence in our lives that it becomes clear that an outside force is influencing our behavior in a positive way.

≫ Do you think God is reluctant to give His Holy Spirit? What insights did Jesus reveal on this matter in John 3:34?

What an incredible statement: "God gives the Spirit without limit." When you seek God's influence in your life, you are not attempting to persuade Him to do something He doesn't want to do. Giving the Spirit pleases God so fully that Jesus said the Father set no limits.

Even with God's Spirit working in your life, you can still take actions that limit His work in you. Even with God's power available to you, you can limit your access to that power and end up with a life out of control. You can resist the Holy Spirit as the religious leaders did during Jesus' ministry on this earth and continued to do after His resurrection and ascension. Read Acts 7:51-53 to see how Stephen rebuked those leaders.

≫ What did Stephen say about these religious leaders?

≫ How could your actions resist God's Holy Spirit? Be specific.

Be filled with the Holy Spirit and be willing to allow the Holy Spirit to have control. Evaluate your life and see if you are doing anything that may be blocking the Holy Spirit from filling you or working in your life. Sometimes a stubborn attitude can block the Spirit's work. You must invite Him to work without limit in every area of your life. Full control depends on being completely influenced by the Spirit!

> According to Romans 8:15-16, what level of intimacy do you have with God? What can you call Him?

> According to this passage, what does God's Holy Spirit say to your human spirit?

As incredible as it sounds, you are God's child. Although you were at one time God's enemy (see Colossians 1:21), now you are a child of God. This gives you status. It is an honor and a privilege. Since you have been adopted into God's family, you must live in a manner consistent with your spiritual heritage.

Father God, I want to be filled with Your Holy Spirit in every area of my life to bring my life under Your complete control.

Lord, help me to always be on guard, and keep me from doing anything that will hinder the work of the Holy Spirit in my life.

DAY 3: *Power Through God's Spirit*

When our lives spin out of control, we can usually hold things together through our personal energy and discipline for a time. However, after a while the stress will become too great and that's when we lose control. We need a source of power that is sufficient to counteract the negative stresses in our lives. God *is* that source of power. The Holy Spirit in you is the means for releasing that power in your life. Jesus promised that when the Holy Spirit works in your life, you receive His power.

➤ Is it appropriate to expand the promise in Acts 1:8 to include other areas of your life besides being a witness for Christ? Why or why not?

➤ What did Paul pray for in Ephesians 3:16?

➤ Write Ephesians 3:20-21 in your own words.

Paul experienced God's power in his own life and prayed that other Christians would experience that power as well. God's power is available for all areas of your life through His Holy Spirit!

➤ What was Paul's warning to the church in Ephesians 4:3?

➤ How could your actions grieve God's Spirit (see Ephesians 4:30)? Be specific.

➤ If you experienced the kind of power promised in Ephesians 3:20, what impact would that power have in your life?

➤ How would you know God had given you that power?

➤ What areas of your life would change? Be specific.

Lord, help me to experience the power of Your Holy Spirit and live under Your control.

Father God, I pray that I will live my life in a manner that is pleasing to You and not settle for less power for living than You intend for me to have.

DAY 4: *No Longer Controlled by Sin*

Without Christ, we are slaves to sin. Slaves have no control over their own lives because they live at the mercy of their master.

➤ How does Paul describe himself in Romans 7:14?

➤ Explain what Paul is saying about his sinful nature in verse 15.

Paul described himself as a slave, but in Christ we have freedom from sin's control. A new source of spiritual power enables you to break free and live.

➣ According to Romans 8:9, what makes it possible for you to no longer be enslaved to sin?

➣ If the Holy Spirit does not live in you, what is your spiritual condition?

Without God's Holy Spirit, you are not Christian. Without the Spirit, you cannot break free from sin's grip on your life. Since the Holy Spirit broke the chains of your slavery to sin, you now have the power to live without gratifying your sinful desires.

➣ What does Galatians 5:16-18 say about the sinful nature and the Holy Spirit?

➣ Explain the choice you must make according to Galatians 6:8.

➣ Paul warned the Thessalonians to be careful about putting out the Holy Spirit's fire. Explain what he meant in 1 Thessalonians 5:19.

➤ How could your own actions put out the Spirit's fire? Be specific.

Keep the fire of the Holy Spirit burning in your life. Let Him take control of your sinful nature. The Spirit provides the power you need to break free from sin. You must choose to cooperate with His leadership in your life. You must make choices and order your life according to His principles. To do so insures that you will enjoy truly abundant life.

Dear God, help me to live today with Your power so that I may sow actions and thoughts that lead to spiritual life and growth.

Lord, help me keep the fire of Your Spirit burning in my life so that I am no longer controlled by my sinful nature.

DAY 5: *Spiritual Character Through the Holy Spirit*

God is building your life from the inside out. As you mature spiritually, He also enables you to mature emotionally. Spiritual strength combined with emotional maturity makes it possible for you to live a controlled life over an extended period of time.

➤ Why do you think Paul referred to the qualities described in Galatians 5:22-23 as "fruit of the Spirit"?

These spiritual and emotional character qualities are the natural product of the Holy Spirit's presence in your life—just like fruit is the natural product of a fruit tree. Use the following chart to evaluate and rank the development of the fruit of the Spirit in your own life. Rate the amount of each quality with 1 representing the degree to which you do *not* see this quality in your life, and 5 representing the degree to which you *do* see this quality in your life. When you identify an area that needs further development, ask God to produce more of that fruit in you through His Holy Spirit.

The Holy Spirit's Fruit in My Life   Scale

Love: my expression of 1 Corinthians 13	1	2	3	4	5
Joy: my response to God's presence in my life	1	2	3	4	5
Peace: my confidence in God's power	1	2	3	4	5
Patience: my willingness to give people time	1	2	3	4	5
Kindness: my sensitivity to others' needs	1	2	3	4	5
Goodness: my desire to do what is good	1	2	3	4	5
Faithfulness: my commitment to keep my word	1	2	3	4	5
Gentleness: my sensitive compassion with people	1	2	3	4	5
Self-control: my discipline under Christ's control	1	2	3	4	5

➤ Write Galatians 5:24-26 in your own words.

In Christ you have all you need to live a life of positive control. You simply need to learn more about the work the Holy Spirit is doing in you so that you can keep in step with Him.

Lord, help me to keep the fire of Your Spirit burning in my life so that I am no longer controlled by my sinful nature.

Heavenly Father, give me the will to let the Holy Spirit do His work without restriction in my life.

DAY 6: *Reflections*

This week's Bible study focused on the Holy Spirit's power in our lives. The only limitations of the Holy Spirit are the ones we put there ourselves. Even with God's power available to us, we can limit our access to that power and end up with a life out of control.

In this study, you have read several verses that illustrate the three ways you limit the power of the Holy Spirit in your life. Examine your actions and motives of the past week. Have you resisted, grieved or put out the fire of the Holy Spirit by any of your actions or attitudes? If yes, then think of ways to put those attitudes out of your life. Let the Holy Spirit work without any restrictions in your life.

Negative feelings about the Holy Spirit's work can lead to strongholds that get in the way of having abundant life. Read 2 Corinthians 10:5 for a biblical definition of a stronghold. Basically, anything that exalts itself in your mind, pretending to be bigger or more powerful than God, becomes a stronghold.

In 2 Corinthians 10:4 you will find that you have the weapons to fight the strongholds. Your weapons are the Word of God and prayer. In combination, these two divinely powered weapons give you the ability to demolish any stronghold that threatens to come in and choke the work of the Holy Spirit in your life.

For more information on prayer using Scripture, read Beth Moore's book *Praying God's Word*.[1] You will be learning about praying Scripture in each of the First Place Bible studies.

The following Scripture prayers will help you get a good start toward memorizing Scripture:

Lord, Your Word is clear that those who are self-seeking and who reject the truth and follow evil will experience Your wrath and anger (see Romans 2:8).[2]

Father, when I sin against You and choose to walk in deception rather than truth, please send others to gently instruct and confront me. Grant me repentance, leading me to a knowledge of the truth (see 2 Timothy 2:25).[3]

How long will I turn Your glory into shame, O Lord? How long will I love delusions and seek false gods? Expose the delusions and false gods in my life, O Lord, and set me free (see Psalm 4:2).

DAY 7: *Reflections*

All you have learned about God's Spirit in this week's study has direct application to your work in the First Place program. Ask God to show you how He wants to deal with your problems. Whether the problems concern food, exercise, prayer, Bible study and/or relationships, God wants to help you take care of them.

Remember, you are adopted into God's family. You are empowered by His Spirit. How could it ever be appropriate for you to live a life out of control? As a child under His control, you must live by the Spirit. The power of the Spirit will help you make the changes you need to improve your life and overcome any strongholds. Make a commitment that you will not resist the Spirit's work in any area of your life in any way.

Use your prayer journal or any small notebook to write down Scriptures such as the ones from the Bible study this week. Memorize them along with your Bible verse for the week. Then use these Scriptures to pray like Jesus did in the wilderness. This will help you to defeat your greatest enemy, Satan.

In the coming weeks you will learn more about Scripture memory and how to use it in your prayer life. Scripture prayers are given at the end of each lesson as examples to help you personalize your own chosen Scriptures into prayers.

Father, You did not give me a spirit that makes me a slave again to fear, but You gave me the Spirit of sonship so that I may call You "Abba, Father" (see Romans 8:15).

Heavenly Father, help me to get rid of all bitterness, rage, anger, brawling and slander, along with every form of malice. Help me to be kind and compassionate to others, forgiving them just as in Christ You forgave me (see Ephesians 4:31-32).

O God of hope, fill me with all joy and peace as I trust in You, so I may overflow with hope by the power of the Holy Spirit (see Romans 15:13).

Notes
1. Beth Moore, *Praying God's Word* (Nashville, TN: Broadman and Holman Publishers, 2000).
2. Ibid., p. 80.
3. Ibid., p. 81.

Group Prayer Requests   Today's Date:_____

Name	Request	Results

THOUGHTS UNDER CONTROL

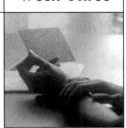

MEMORY VERSE

Finally, brothers, whatever is true, whatever is noble, whatever is right, whatever is pure, whatever is lovely, whatever is admirable—if anything is excellent or praiseworthy—think about such things.

Philippians 4:8

A little boy described thinking this way: "Thinking is when your mouth stays shut and your head keeps talking to itself." Psychologists estimate 10,000 thoughts go through a person's mind each day. If the little boy and the psychologists are right, your mind is having an incredible conversation with itself! Since what you think impacts what you do, you must discipline your thoughts. Only when your thoughts are under control can you keep your life under control.

In this week's study, you'll learn how to screen your thoughts, so what you think will steer your life in a positive direction. The memory verse gives a practical plan for getting thoughts under control. Using eight keywords, Paul created a mental screen for filtering out destructive thoughts.

DAY 1: *Only What Is True and Noble*

Ralph Waldo Emerson once said, "Beware of what you set your mind on for that you will surely become." Christians committed to becoming like Christ must control their thoughts.

You cannot afford to allow thoughts to race through your mind like an undisciplined preschooler. You must assume responsibility for your thoughts.

➤ Read 1 Corinthians 14:20. What does the phrase "in your thinking be adults" mean to you?

God never commands you in Scripture to do anything that you can-not do—with His help. If God says, "Think about such things," that means you are able to make choices and exercise control over those thoughts.

⇒ What is the warning found in Romans 13:14?

Use the following information to form a working definition for what is true and what is noble:

Definition

True means that which is in accordance with fact and agrees with reality; real, genuine, authentic.

Noble means showing high moral qualities, ideas or greatness of character; grand, stately.

Scripture

⇒ **True:** John 8:14; Romans 3:4. What do these verses say about being true?

⇒ **Noble:** 1 Timothy 3:8,11. What do these verses say about being noble?

Commentators

True: Lenski says, "True in the Bible refers to something that is spiri-tually true, not lying."[1]

Noble: *Tyndale Concise Bible Commentary* uses "honorable, dignified or elevated."[2]
Barclay refers to that which has the "dignity of holiness upon it."[3]

The Opposite of . . .

True is what is false from God's perspective.

Noble is what is crude, crass or vulgar.

Based on these ideas, write your own definition of each of the following:

➤ True:

➤ Noble:

How difficult it is to screen thoughts that are crass, crude or false. Without careful attention, you can clutter your mind with so much that is silly and worthless that you lose your capacity to focus on valuable thoughts. One writer has said, "Satan loves to use vacant minds as dumping grounds." What applies to vacant minds applies to minds littered with mental debris. You must post "No dumping" signs in your mind to insure that you maintain your ability to think about spiritual truths.

Heavenly Father, fill my thoughts and mind today with only the true and noble thoughts that will keep me focused on You.

Father God, help me today to see what is true and noble about You, others and myself.

DAY 2: *Only What Is Right*

You face an incredible challenge today as you seek to determine what is right and to do it while the world tells you that nothing is inherently right or wrong. Against the world's subjective ethics, you must stand as a person who says "There is right, and there is wrong—God has told me."

The battle for your mind is a spiritual battle. You must choose each day to take your thoughts captive to make them obedient to Christ.

➤ According to 2 Corinthians 10:5, what is involved in making your thoughts obedient to Christ?

➤ What role do right thoughts play in the day-to-day spiritual battle?

So many times Christians find themselves in situations where their thoughts may not be pleasing and right to God. Temptations cause every Christian to think thoughts that are not right. Only the Holy Spirit can help you fight the battle and bring your thoughts back to obedience to Him.

Thoughts of revenge or retaliation against someone who has hurt you are not right. If they come only for a fleeting moment but then give way to thoughts on how you can forgive, you are allowing the Spirit to control your thoughts. Satan has no defense against God's offense. Let's look at information you can use to form a working definition of "right."

Definition

Right means being in conformity with moral law, standards or truth.

Scripture

Right is often used in connection with the word "just" and tied to your standing before God and His character. In this context, it seems to apply to what is considered just through God's evaluation.

Commentators

Barclay says it was "the word of duty faced and duty done."[3] Others have commented that "right" applied to what should be done to please God in a particular situation.

The Opposite of . . .

Right is what is wrong or inappropriate from God's perspective.

➤ Write your personal working definition of the word "right" that you will use to determine if a thought is acceptable to God.

Thoughts that cause you to stray from God's will or what God deems to be right become sin when they are not checked. Whenever questionable thoughts come into your mind, ask yourself if the results of the thoughts would be pleasing to God. No one else knows your thoughts but God.

➤ What does Hebrews 4:12 tell you about your thoughts?

God reveals to you through His Word what is right and what is wrong. You have no excuse not to know. The truth is clearly evident in the Bible.

Holy Lord God, help me to stand firm in my faith and keep my thoughts under Your control.

Dear Jesus, discipline my mind to focus on what is right rather than what is popular at the moment.

DAY 3: *Only What Is Pure*

Like a polluted river, our minds can become clogged with impurity. Without diligence, the normal course of our lives brings so much that is impure into our minds that we can become stagnant in our thinking. Once impurity settles into our minds, we can easily dwell on those negative thoughts; and without strong corrective actions, a steady focus on impure thoughts will send our lives out of control. Our best action is to monitor the purity of our thoughts.

Remember David? When his eyes focused on the beauty of Bathsheba, his thoughts became impure and he wanted her. He then allowed Satan to gain control of those thoughts which led to sin. In the following chart, read each type of entertainment or information and then determine how it can be the source of impure thoughts.

Media	Impact on Your Thoughts
Television programs	_____
Radio	_____
Music	_____
Books	_____
Magazines or newspapers	_____
Movies (whether theater, video or TV)	_____
The Internet	_____

The media can also be a source of information and impact us for good. Evaluate what you read, watch and listen to by God's standards. Today you have a choice of a wide variety of inspirational reading in both fiction and nonfiction. Inspirational messages are available from various churches across the country through television and radio. The computer can be a valuable source for information and for keeping in touch by e-mail with missionaries, friends and family. The forms of media are not impure in themselves; the impurity comes from what people do with them.

Now you can form a working definition of what is pure.

Definition

Pure means free from anything that taints, impairs or infects.

Scripture

➤ What do 2 Corinthians 11:2; Titus 2:5 and 1 John 3:3 say about purity?

Commentators

Barclay said that in a ceremonial sense "pure" described what had been cleansed so that it was fit to be brought into God's presence.[4]

The Opposite of . . .

Pure is polluted and unacceptable.

➤ Write your personal working definition of the word "pure" that you will use to determine if your thoughts are acceptable to God.

➤ What does Proverbs 15:26 say about the thoughts of the wicked in contrast to the thoughts of the pure?

➤ In light of what you have learned today, would you want the contents of your thoughts during the past week to be broadcast at a church service next Sunday? Why or why not?

As you have learned with David, even those who are committed to God battle with impure thoughts. You must be determined to fight and win the battle for pure thinking one thought at a time.

 Heavenly Father, purify my mind and keep it free from anything that can pollute it.

DAY 4: *Only What Is Lovely or Admirable*

Loveliness usually brings to mind beauty, but it refers to more than just physical beauty. Have you ever seen someone who may not necessarily be beautiful by the world's standards but is nonetheless described as lovely. The person probably has a certain spirit of graciousness and sweetness that comes from deep inside and can't help but shine through to others. If we look at the world around us through God's eyes, we will see what is lovely and worthy of our enjoyment.

Things that are admirable inspire us. Seeing a person overcome sin and come to Jesus should inspire us and bring about thoughts of God's love. We see the power of God in a person who lives through a time of difficulty strengthened by God's grace and love, living a life worthy of admiration and respect. Be careful about your selection of things or persons to admire. Only those things that are God honoring are worthy to be admired.

Now study the information you can use to form working definitions of "lovely" and "admirable."

Definition

> **Lovely** means having those qualities that inspire love or affection; morally or spiritually attractive.

> **Admirable** means inspiring or deserving of esteem.

Scripture

> **Lovely:** only used in Philippians 4:8.

> **Admirable:** only used in Philippians 4:8.

Commentators

> **Lovely:** The focus is on things that would be inspiring to others if they were to hear them.

> Barclay wrote that "winsome is the best translation," referring to "that which calls forth love."[5]

> **Admirable:** In the *King James Version* the original Greek word is translated as "of good report."

The Opposite of . . .

Lovely is repulsive.

Admirable is negative or depressing.

➣ Write your personal working definition of each word so that you will be able to use them to determine if your thoughts are acceptable to God.

Lovely:

Admirable:

You have the choice. You can fill your mind with things that inspire and build up, that are lovely and attractive or you can fill it with the repulsive, negative thoughts. When God is in control, your thoughts will be those that will inspire you and cause you to enjoy the beauty and loveliness of God's world.

➣ How does Psalm 84:1-2 relate to this week's memory verse?

Father God, fill my mind with thoughts that focus on positive things, on possibilities, on potential.

Lord God, direct my soul and heart to focus on You and the beauty of Your world.

DAY 5: *Only What Is Excellent and Praiseworthy*

In the 1980s a book titled *In Search of Excellence* became a best-seller. The authors searched for companies in America that operated with higher standards than others and were unwilling to compromise and settle for mediocrity. How tragic that excellence in business was so unusual that it attracted attention. Unfortunately, the same problem would exist if a search were launched to find people whose minds were filled with excellent thoughts.

What is excellent *is* worthy of praise. Ultimately you live your life in the presence of God and His evaluation must be the measure of your success. You know of your need to praise God, but are you living your life in such a way that God can praise you?

When you allow mediocrity to fill your mind and accept that which is second best, your thoughts turn to those things that are not up to God's standards. Set your standards high, beginning with the way you think.

A great place to begin is Psalm 8. The *King James Version* uses the word "excellent" for the word translated "majestic" in the *New International Version*.

➻ How could Psalm 8 help you focus on the excellence of God?

Let's take a look at information you can use to develop a working definition of "excellent" and "praiseworthy."

Definition

Excellent means outstandingly good among its kind, of exceptional merit.

Praiseworthy means commendable.

Scripture

Excellent: used only in Paul's writings.

Praiseworthy: Greek word as translated in Philippians 4:8 is not used elsewhere.

Commentators

Excellent: In classical writing, the word described every kind of excellence.

Praiseworthy: *Tyndale Concise Bible Commentary* says the word refers to something that deserves praise or calls down praise from God.[6]

The Opposite of . . .

Excellent is common, mediocre, mundane.
Praiseworthy is worthy of condemnation.

➤ What standard have you set for your life? Check the following statements that you may have said at one time or another either at work or in general with your life:

- ☐ This is good enough—not great, but good enough.
- ☐ If they want better work, they should pay me more!
- ☐ What are you, some sort of perfectionist? My work is fine.

Statements such as these *could* indicate problems. Is there a possibility you might be settling for mediocrity?

➤ What would your life or job be like if you set high standards and were able to declare: "This is my best work; I'm proud to put my name on it"?

➤ Write your own personal definitions for "excellent" and "praiseworthy."

Excellent:

Praiseworthy:

Heavenly Father, You alone are worthy of my praise. Fill me with Your glory and bring my thoughts under Your control.

Father God, help me to set high standards in the way that I think and work, so You will be pleased.

DAY 6: *Reflections*

In this week's study, we have learned what kinds of thoughts are pleasing to God. By focusing your thinking on the things set forth in Philippians 4:8, you fill your mind with those things that bring pleasure to God and affect your own life and the lives of those around you in positive ways.

One way to keep your thoughts centered on what is true, noble, pure, excellent, praiseworthy, right, lovely and admirable is to memorize God's Word and think on those words that lead you to worship God. Satan cannot get a foothold when your mind is filled with Scripture. Scripture and right thinking crowd him out, leaving room only for God. Strongholds cannot stand against the Word of God. The walls are weakened and eventually fall completely when your mind is filled with the Holy Spirit and Scripture.

Here then is another reason for memorizing Scripture: to fill your thoughts with what is pleasing to God. No situation will be too difficult and no temptation will be so great that Scriptures cannot help you through it successfully.

You probably know the basics concerning the work of Satan, but do you really consider him your enemy? Until you do, you won't put up a defense strong enough to defeat him. Your enemy is just waiting for you to let down your guard. Remember 1 John 4:4; only God is greater than the one who is in the world.

Use the following Scripture prayer as you pray for victory over your enemy, Satan:

Father God, may the words of my mouth and the meditations of my heart always be pleasing in Your sight, for You are my Rock and my Redeemer (see Psalm 19:14).

O Lord, I know You have searched me and know me when I sit or when I rise and You perceive my thoughts from afar. Keep my thoughts focused on You and fill me with Your Holy Spirit (see Psalm 139:1-2).

"Search me, O God, and know my heart; test me and know my anxious thoughts. See if there is any offensive way in me, and lead me in the way everlasting" (Psalm 139:23-24).

DAY 7: *Reflections*

In her book *Praying God's Word*, Beth Moore says that churches tend to give the devil either far too much credit or not nearly enough. In addition, Satan has successfully duped the vast majority of churches into imbalance regarding all things concerning or threatening him.[7]

We are seeing rampant wickedness and evil in the world today. We find that places that were once places of safety are now places of violence. Churches and schools are no longer havens where parents take their children with confidence that they will be safe. Columbine High School and Wedgwood Baptist Church became known nationwide, not because of their excellence as a school or church, but because of the violence unleashed by Satan. Be assured, Satan is alive and well and making his presence known.

Your defense against evil is to be steeped in the Word of God. Sin crouches at your door just waiting to devour you (see Genesis 4:7). You must arm yourself for the battle that rages all around you. Pursue the heart of God and all things concerning Him. Think on God and the things set forth by Paul as those things that will be pleasing to God.

Use the following prayers for those times when you know or even suspect Satan is working to defeat you. You have inherited the right to victory—claim it.

 Who is like Your children, O God, a people saved by the Lord? You are my shield and helper and my glorious sword. Cause my enemy to cower, Lord! Trample down his high places (see Deuteronomy 33:29).[8]

Lord God, I will shout for joy when You make me victorious, and I will lift up a banner in the name of my God! Please, Lord, grant these requests (see Psalm 20:5).[9]

Father, help me to understand that Satan, the ultimate thief, comes only to steal and kill and destroy; You came so that I could have life and have it more abundantly (see John 10:10).[10]

Heavenly Father, keep my thoughts on whatever is true, whatever is noble, whatever is right, whatever is pure, whatever is lovely, whatever is admirable; if anything is excellent or praiseworthy, let me think about it (see Philippians 4:8).

Notes

1. R.C.H. Lenski, *The Interpretation of St. Paul's Epistles to the Galatians, to the Ephesians and to the Phillipians* (Columbus, OH: Lutheran Book Concern, 1937), n.p.
2. Robert B. Hughes and J. Carl Laney, *Tyndale Concise Bible Commentary* (Wheaton, IL: Tyndale House Publishers, 2001), n.p.
3. William Barclay, *The Letters to the Galatians and Ephesians* (Philadelphia: Westminster Press, 1976), n.p.
4. Ibid.
5. Ibid.
6. Hughes and Laney, *Tyndale Concise Bible Commentary*, n.p.
7. Beth Moore, *Praying God's Word* (Nashville, TN: Broadman and Holman Publishers, 2000), p. 309.
8. Ibid., p. 313.
9. Ibid., p. 316.
10. Ibid., p. 326.

GROUP PRAYER REQUESTS   TODAY'S DATE:_____

NAME	REQUEST	RESULTS

ACTIONS UNDER CONTROL

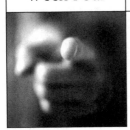

MEMORY VERSE

I have been crucified with Christ and I no longer live,
but Christ lives in me. The life I live in the body,
I live by faith in the Son of God, who loved me
and gave Himself for me.
Galatians 2:20

When life slips out of control, it's always possible to find a reason—usually a reason that shifts the blame to other people or situations. Here are a few examples:

- He made me do it.
- She's to blame.
- The temptation was too strong.
- It caught me at a weak moment.
- I didn't think it could happen to me.

In this week's study you'll learn more about God's expectation for your actions. You'll discover how God equips you to keep your actions under His control.

DAY 1: *Shifting of Blame*

From the beginning—the *very* beginning—people have struggled to keep their lives under control. The book of Genesis tells how the first two people responded after they lost control of their lives.

➤ In Genesis 3:8-13, God asked Adam and Eve to explain their actions. How did they respond?

Given the opportunity, most people attempt to shift the blame when confronted with sin. Adam's response was especially interesting since it seems he was attempting to place the blame on God because He had given Eve to him! The pattern set in the beginning continues.

➻ In what ways do you tend to shift blame rather than assume responsibility for your actions? Be specific.

God created us in His image and gave us the freedom to make moral choices. He holds us responsible for the choices we make. Blame shifting is not an option; we are accountable to God for our actions.

The primary decision for which we are all responsible is what we decide to do regarding Jesus' offer of salvation. God works in the hearts of all people, drawing them to seek and receive Christ. Only in Christ is the powerful grip of sin broken. Once we become Christians, we die to sin's domination. Christ takes up residence in our lives. Through His powerful life in us, we are enabled to resist and overcome the drive to sin.

➻ What is the common idea presented in both Romans 6:2 and Galatians 5:24?

The image is that we were slaves to sin, controlled and dominated. Only through death could we find release. However, through Christ's death for us, liberation from sin becomes an option. In spiritual terms, we can die and then live again through Christ. So complete is the new life Christ gives us, we can count our former selves as dead to the old life.

➻ What does Romans 6:11 say about sin and death?

≫ A slave owner cannot control a dead slave. The Christian life is your declaration of freedom. Since sin can no longer dominate your life when you become a Christian, what force should control your life?

As slaves of righteousness, we can live a life that pleases God. The age of negative domination ends; the age of positive spiritual control begins.

If you have trusted Christ as your Savior, you are set free from sin's suffocating control. If you are not a Christian, open your life to Christ. Talk to your First Place leader and find out how to trust the One who can give you freedom from sin. That is the most important choice for which you are responsible. Once you accept Christ, the Holy Spirit will come dwell in you and help you to control the temptations that will come into your life.

Heavenly Father, I put my trust in You as my Savior and Lord. Thank You for sending Your Son to die for my sin.

Lord God, though my body be a slave to sin, give me the freedom that only Christ can give to those who trust in Him as Savior.

DAY 2: *Foundation for Life Control*

You have three primary steps to take to bring your actions under Christ's control. These steps are described in Romans 6:11-13. Although the principles sound somewhat abstract, they lay a solid foundation of spiritual truth from which you can work.

≫ What is the first step as explained in Romans 6:11?

≫ What is the second principle for control as found in Romans 6:12?

➣ What should you offer to God according to Romans 6:13?

When you count yourself dead to sin, you simply remind yourself that you no longer have to respond to sin's demands. When ideas or thoughts push you toward sinful action, you do not have to respond. You have choices because of Jesus Christ. Sin has no authority, no irresistible influence in your life. You are free!

Since you are dead to sin, it naturally follows that you should not let sin reign in your life. Having broken free from the tyrant, why would you invite the tyrant back in?

Imagine yourself in a situation in which you are tempted to act in a way that will displease God. How could you use the three principles in Romans 6:11-13 to choose actions that would please God?

➣ Principle 1: Count myself as dead to sin.

➣ Principle 2: Do not let sin reign in my life.

➣ Principle 3: Offer every part of my life to God.

In spite of all God has done to empower you to keep your life under control, you may still find yourself failing, still sinning. Fortunately, God provides what you need once life slips out of control. The Bible clearly states that people will sin even after they become Christians. Sin is not God's design, and yet sin continues.

✎ Explain 1 John 1:8 in your own words.

✎ Explain 1 John 1:10 in your own words.

If there are unconfessed sins in your life, confess them now. Agree with God in His assessment of your actions. He will strengthen you to walk with greater victory over sin in the future.

 Thank You, Father God, for providing what I need when my life spins out of control and forgiving me when I let sin control me.

Jesus, give me the strength I need to follow You to greater victory over sin.

DAY 3: *Control of Temptation*

Even armed with spiritual truth, situations develop that push Christians to the limits. At times, sin's attraction and temptation's enticement feel too powerful to resist. You learned in the first week that even a man of God like David gave in to temptation. When you give in to temptation, your life spins out of control. Remind yourself of the truth of Romans 6:11-13 and you will reinforce your resistance.

Read 1 Corinthians 10:13. Here you will find an explanation of the five things you need to know about resisting temptation.

Study the principles presented in the following chart. Think of a particular temptation you face and explain how you could use each principle to resist that temptation.

Temptation Principles	How I Can Use This Principle
1 Temptation is common.	
2 God is faithful.	
3 The limits are set.	
4 There's always a way out.	
5 You can stand the pressure.	

Think of the promises in 1 Corinthians 10:13. We are all tempted, but God is faithful because He will not allow us to be tempted beyond what we can resist and He will make a way out of the temptation.

God knows your limits and always provides a way for you to win over temptation. He can help you experience the reality of these temptation principles today.

Take a few minutes and consider all that Christ has done for you. He endured the agony of the Cross to set you free from sin. His grace has given you a new life. He promises to always be with you through the Holy Spirit who lives in you. The best thanks you can give God is to live your life in His control.

✎ What are two practical ways you could say thank You to Him by the way you live today?

1.

2.

✎ How could you use your efforts in the First Place program as an expression of thanks to God for all He has done for you?

 Father God, help me to live today in a way that would be an appropriate expression of gratitude for what You have done for me.

Thank You, Father, for providing a way for temptation to never overpower my life. I praise You for providing a way for me to escape the snares of temptation.

DAY 4: *Control in Times of Weakness*

As you battle to keep your life under Christ's control, there are times when you may feel very weak. Sin's unrelenting assault against your life creates spiritual fatigue. In desperation, you may cry out for help and strength.

Should you seek to keep your life under control simply to avoid negative consequences? No. You have a far more important reason—to honor Christ with your life.

⇒ What common idea is contained in both Ephesians 4:1 and Colossians 1:10?

Your motivation for Christian living isn't fear of God's punishment or a frantic drive to earn God's favor. Christ paid for your sin through His death and extended the benefits of salvation to us through His grace.

⇒ How would you summarize the lesson Paul speaks of in 2 Corinthians 12:8-10?

The good news is that God hears your cry. When you are weak, He will make you strong. He will use the weakest area in your life as a platform from which to exhibit His power. He promises never to leave you or forsake you.

The following verses reveal principles about God's power in your life. After you read each passage, write the central idea of that Scripture.

⇒ Romans 4:20-21

⇒ Ephesians 3:20

⇒ Ephesians 6:10

≫ Colossians 1:29

≫ 2 Peter 1:3

When you are weak, God will make you strong. Call on Him to deliver you from all sin and temptation. He is faithful and will stand by you and see you through all your deep valleys.

 Heavenly Father, thank You for giving me strength to face the struggles that come into my life and threaten to overcome me. Lord Jesus, help me to live my life under Your control.

DAY 5: *Control Through Spiritual Caution*

Prominent Christian men may sometimes find themselves in difficult situations when they work with the public. Billy Graham, the great evangelist, once said, "My greatest fear is that I'll do something or say something that will bring disrepute on the gospel of Christ." Graham is known for cautious humility. An example of this is found in a reported description of how he guards against sexual sin: No male on the Graham staff is ever alone in a room with a female unless the door is kept open. Graham never enters a hotel room until it has been checked by an aide. And he never opens his hotel room door unless he knows for sure who is on the other side. Is Billy Graham paranoid? No, he's simply realistic about the power of sin—or even the appearance of sin—and the battle Christians must wage to resist sin's pull.

The following Scriptures explain the importance of living with spiritual caution. Write a principle from each verse that you could use in your life.

➻ 1 Corinthians 10:12

➻ Ephesians 5:11-12

➻ Hebrews 2:1

➻ After reading 1 Corinthians 8:9, write one way your careless actions can have a negative impact on others.

➻ What is the warning in 1 Peter 5:8?

In spite of all the cautions you take, you may find yourself giving in to temptation. Once you sin, the Bible says you must confess that sin. Confession of sin means to admit to God that a particular action or thought is indeed sin. Once you agree with God that your actions are sinful, He forgives you.

➻ What does 1 John 1:9 mean to you?

Confession of sin brings about forgiveness and reconciliation. You will renew your mind when your focus is turned to God and you have filled your mind with His Word. Write the memory verse for this week in your own words.

➤ Galatians 2:20

As you complete this week's study, consider what Paul wrote in 2 Corinthians 6:3 about not being a stumbling block to others or careless about your witness.

➤ How can Paul's warning and teaching be applied to your efforts in the First Place program?

Instead of being a stumbling block, be an encourager this week. Drop a note by mail or e-mail, or call a fellow group member and encourage him or her in the First Place program. In addition, pray for the members of your group in your daily prayer time. Write their requests in your prayer journal.

Heavenly Father, help me to keep my thoughts focused on You so that I will neither give in to my own temptations nor become a stumbling block for anyone else.

Father God, I am Your humble servant. Forgive my failures and restore my relationship with You. Hold me fast and keep me from drifting away from Your truths.

DAY 6: Reflections

This week's Bible study instructs you on how to keep your actions under control. People who know you are a Christian will be watching your actions. Remember, you no longer live in the flesh, Christ lives in you, and you live by the faith God gave you through His Son, Jesus Christ. As Peter warned, you must always be self-controlled and alert because Satan is busy looking for your weak spots.

In his book *In Touch with God*, Charles Stanley wrote:

> I am so glad Jesus did not outsmart Satan in a battle of the minds. I have tried that and failed miserably. I am glad He did not discuss the temptation with Satan and resist him that way. Eve tried that, and she got nowhere. I am glad Jesus did not use raw willpower, though I imagine He could have. My willpower is pretty useless when Satan really turns on the steam. Jesus verbally confronted Satan with the truth and eventually, Satan gave up and left. God's Word takes you right to the heart of the matter. It allows you to see things for what they really are.[1]

If you filter all temptation through the truth in God's Word, Satan will lose the battle every time. He cannot stand under the pressure of truth. Satan is the god of lies, distortion, rationalization and blame. When you hide God's Word in your heart and pray for guidance from the Holy Spirit, Satan shudders with horror and flees.

At first, memorizing all 10 verses for this study may seem like an impossible task. However, if you memorize one each week and continue to repeat each verse each week, you will soon have all 10 verses memorized. The secret is to make each verse yours and use it when you need help with the situations or temptations that come. No matter how many other verses you choose to memorize, always make it your goal to memorize the week's verse.

Here are a few verses you can memorize and recite as prayers to help you resist the temptations Satan puts in your path.

Lord God, keep me from conforming to this world. Transform me by the renewing of my mind that I may prove what is the good and pleasing and perfect will of God (see Romans 12:2).

Heavenly Father, thank You for arming me with strength for the battle and subduing my adversaries (see Psalm 18:39).

Lord Jesus, You promised that sin would not be my master because I am not under the law but under Your grace (see Romans 6:14).

I know that if this earthly house, this tent, is destroyed, I have a building from You, an eternal house not made by human hands (see 2 Corinthians 5:1).

DAY 7: *Reflections*

A stronghold in your life may cause you to stumble and give in to temptation. God is more powerful than any stronghold you have in your life. Whether that stronghold involves poor eating habits, relationships with others, your rebellious spirit, pride or feelings of guilt, God can overcome it. He sent the Holy Spirit to give you power over your strongholds.

God equips you with His Word and with prayer to bring under submission any unhealthy or sinful desires you may have. He wants to change your sinful habits and desires to those that pursue His grace and build you up. God's desire is for you to be successful in all your endeavors that are according to His will for your life.

In your prayer journal, remember to write down Scriptures you find to be helpful reminders of God's love and grace. Keep a list of prayer requests weekly and pray for those on the list each day. A serendipity of memorizing Scripture is finding you have an appropriate passage that applies to a friend's prayer request or even a need of your own.

When Beth Moore speaks of strongholds, she makes it clear that strongholds are not a problem limited to unbelievers. Many Christians are under the impression that, once saved, they will no longer be bothered by the temptations of their old lives. If only that were true! She reminds you that a stronghold is "anything that steals, kills, or destroys the abundant, fruitful life of a believer."[2]

The first four of the following Scripture prayers are from *Praying God's Word*. The last one is your memory verse.

Test me, O Lord, and try me, examine my heart and my mind; for Your love is ever before me, and I desire to walk continually in Your truth (see Psalm 26:2-3).[3]

Teach me Your way, O Lord, and I will walk in Your truth; give me an undivided heart, that I may fear Your name (see Psalm 86:11).[4]

Father, You sent Your Holy Spirit to be a Counselor to me. He came straight from You to me and other believers. He is the Spirit of truth who goes out from the Father, and He faithfully testifies truth to me concerning Your Son, Jesus (see John 15:26).[5]

Father God, You have no greater joy than to know that Your children are walking in the truth (see 3 John 4).[6]

Heavenly Father, I have been crucified with Christ and I no longer live, but Christ lives in me. The life I now live in the body, I live by faith in the Son of God who loved me and gave Himself for me (see Galatians 2:20).

Notes
1. Charles Stanley, *In Touch with God* (Nashville, TN: Thomas Nelson, 1997), n.p.
2. Beth Moore, *Praying God's Word* (Nashville, TN: Broadman and Holman Publishers, 2000). p. 14.
3. Ibid., p. 76.
4. Ibid.
5. Ibid., p. 79.
6. Ibid., p. 83.

GROUP PRAYER REQUESTS   TODAY'S DATE:_____

NAME	REQUEST	RESULTS

DESIRES UNDER CONTROL

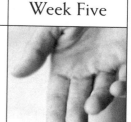

*I have learned the secret of being content
in any and every situation, whether well fed or
hungry whether living in plenty or in want.
I can do everything through him who gives me strength.*
Philippians 4:12-13

A cartoon pictured two mules standing in adjoining pastures of lush green grass, separated by a tightly strung barbed-wire fence. Each mule had poked his head through the fence, and while pressing against the barbs, was attempting to eat the grass in the next pasture. Under the scene, the cartoonist had written one word: "Discontent."

"Discontent" could be defined as the restless desire for something more or different. In a world driven by restless desire, God offers the only antidote: contentment.

In this week's study, you'll examine three negative emotions that fuel discontent: lust, greed and envy. Then you'll learn more about spiritual contentment and how to develop that quality in your life.

DAY 1: *Contentment—Life Under Control*

Desire fuels discontent which may channel itself through lust, greed and/or envy. Once any of these negative emotional drives begins to surge through your life, your life can readily skid out of control. The power of these negative emotions causes you to struggle even more as you try to resist temptation and please God. In reality, these emotions cannot be allowed to reside unchallenged in a Christian's life. Once entrenched, they reap havoc.

When you can think of yesterday without regret and tomorrow without fear, you are near true contentment. Such insight resonates with spiritual truth. In Philippians 4:11-12, Paul describes his personal experience of contentment. Summarize the key ideas in each verse.

⟫ Verse 11:

⟫ Verse 12:

Is it possible to be content no matter what circumstances you experience? In his life, Paul had faced incredible obstacles, far more than most Christians would ever encounter. Yet in each situation, he tested one simple idea: If I have Christ, will I have all I need? Over and over again, whether in want or in plenty, he found that Christ is enough. Toward the end of his life when he wrote the Philippian letter, Paul stated with confidence: Christ is enough!

⟫ In what practical ways would your life change if you could be content in any and every situation? Be specific.

Even the dictionary definition of contentment suggests a spiritual challenge to pursue: happy with what one has or is, not desiring something more or different. In a world marked by churning discontent, the mere suggestion of contentment offers hope.

This week, you'll examine three negative emotions that breed discontent. Write your own definition for each of the following words:

Lust:

Greed:

Envy:

Repeat the memory verse in some way: Say it to another person, write it on a memo, send it in a message to a member of your First Place class or write it in your journal. Let contentment be your focus this week. Find ways in which you can exhibit positive emotions of love and joy.

 Heavenly Father, help me to break the hold of negative emotions and teach me to live with spiritual contentment.

Thank You, Father, that through Your power, I can bring my wants under control.

DAY 2: *Lust—Desire out of Control*

Until we bring lust under control, we will never experience the joy of contentment. "Lust" means a desire to gratify the senses or appetites; to feel an intense desire for something. W. E. Vine noted that in the Bible, the word "lust" denotes strong desire for anything, usually with a negative connotation.[1]

The following charts contain groups of verses. Read each group of verses and then write a summary of the main ideas or common words and phrases contained in them.

Characteristics of Unbelievers	
Ephesians 4:19 1 Thessalonians 4:5 2 Timothy 4:3 Titus 3:3 1 Peter 1:14 2 Peter 3:3	

Evidence of the Sinful Nature	
Ephesians 2:3 Colossians 3:5 James 1:14 1 Peter 2:11 2 Peter 2:18 1 John 2:16	

The Bible describes lust as a primary characteristic of the life of some-one who is not a Christian. Without Christ's control, the sinful nature runs rampant and lust often takes over. After reading the following verses, write a short description of the type of lust each verse mentions:

≫ Matthew 5:28

≫ 1 Timothy 6:9

Lust may be sexual, financial or material possessions. It's even possible for a strong desire for food to be lustful! Whenever your desires begin to control you, rather than you controlling them, you have a problem.

In the first week of this study we looked at David's road to sin. He saw Bathsheba, and he wanted her. His sexual lust for a beautiful woman led him to commit adultery and then arrange a death to cover it up. Just as David's sin compounded, so do ours when we give in to lust.

≫ In 1 Timothy 6:10, what is Timothy's warning to those who would lust after money?

The desire for more money and material possessions is common, even among Christians. Young people go to college and seek careers that will reward them financially. Too many adults go into serious credit card debt to satisfy the lust or desire for possessions and material wealth.

≫ According to 1 Timothy 6:11, what are the things Christians should seek in life?

Lust for wealth and possessions is connected to greed—tomorrow's topic. Later in this study, you will learn how the Bible says you can regain control over your desires.

Heavenly Father, make my strongest desire in life be to know You in a more intimate relationship.

Lord, fill my mind with love, faith and joy with godliness, endurance and gentleness as my goals.

DAY 3: *Greed—Wants out of Control*

Contentment continues to be elusive as long as greed undercuts your satisfaction. "Greed" means an excessive desire for getting or having something, especially wealth; a desire for more than one needs or deserves, wanting or taking all one can get with no thought of others.

Because greed is a negative drive that plagues our lives, it must be brought under control. In fact, the Bible mentions greed, or covetousness, as one of the all-encompassing sins we should battle.

➩ Consider Exodus 20:17; Romans 7:7-8 and 13:9. Based on these passages, how seriously does God take the problem of greed (i.e., covetousness)?

If greed is allowed to grow unchecked in our lives, it will influence the way we treat other people.

➩ According to 1 Thessalonians 2:5 and 2 Peter 2:3,14, how can greed hurt relationships?

➩ Luke 12:13-21 relates Jesus' teaching about greed. In Luke 12:15, what did Jesus say about greed?

Paul confronted greed in the people of the Early Church and wrote warnings to them in his letters.

❧ What is Paul's stern warning in Ephesians 5:5?

❧ What other evils are included with greed in Colossians 3:5-6? What does that tell you about the seriousness of the sin of greed?

❧ How are we to respond to these evils?

Unless you are vigilant, greed can exert its influence in your life. Driven by greed, life can spiral out of control. Only God through His Holy Spirit can free you from the bonds of greed in your life.

 Heavenly Father, grant me contentment and satisfaction in life based on my relationship with You.

Lord God, I pray for freedom from any kind of greed that may come into my life. Help me to keep my eyes focused only on You.

DAY 4: Envy—Comparison out of Control

The Roman philosopher Seneca once said, "Not he who has little, but he who wishes for more is poor." Lust seeks gratification of the senses. Greed wants more, more, more. Envy hates others for perceived advantages. "Envy" means a feeling of discontent and ill will because of another's advantages; a resentful dislike of another who has something that one desires. W. E. Vine wrote that the biblical meaning of the word is "the feeling of displeasure produced by witnessing or hearing of the advantage or prosperity of others; this evil sense always attaches to the word."[2]

Since the focus of envy is people, it is not unusual that others are hurt as a direct result of envy. Read the following Scriptures; then identify who was hurt and how:

➤ Matthew 27:18

➤ Acts 7:9

➤ Acts 13:45

➤ Write the truth of Philippians 4:19 in relation to envy.

In light of this verse, you can see that envy has no place in the life of a Christian. God promises to give you strength (see Philippians 4:13) and meet your needs no matter what situation you face in life. Find your contentment in Him—nowhere else.

The Bible also identifies envy as the characteristic of a person who is not a Christian—one who is dominated by the sinful nature. After reading the following verses, write what each passage tells you about the evil of envy:

➤ Mark 7:21-23

✎ Romans 1:29

✎ Galatians 5:19-21

✎ Titus 3:3

✎ What is the common thread or idea which winds through each of these verses?

Envy undermines any hope of contentment in life. The sin that springs from envy often hurts others. For your own stability in life and for the sake of others, you cannot tolerate envy's lodging within you. It is a spiritual cancer that demands radical surgery.

 Dear Lord, help me to rejoice in the blessings and successes of others and find complete satisfaction in Your blessings for my life.

Father God, remove all evidences of envy from my life so that I might enjoy the freedom of Your perfect will.

DAY 5: *Lust, Greed and Envy Under Control*

As a Christian, nothing in your life is able to hold you as a spiritual hostage. The emotional drives of lust, greed and envy are strong and destructive, yet because of Christ and His power in your life, you can have victory over these negative drives. Consider Philippians 2:13—God will give you the will and the power to do what He asks you to do.

There are practical ways God can help you overcome lust, greed or envy in your life.

→ According to 1 John 2:16-17, what is the result of lust?

→ What does Proverbs 15:27 say about the results of greed?

→ What does Proverbs 14:30 say about the differences between contentment and living with an envious nature?

→ How does Hebrews 13:5 relate to lust, envy or covetousness?

The rich young man in Matthew 19:16-22 mistakenly believed that the wealth he had amassed was his alone. He didn't want to give it up to follow Jesus. Jesus viewed his attitude as a form of greed. When you choose to follow Jesus, you don't have to fret over these matters because He knows your needs and will supply them.

Read the following verses; then write insights and ideas that can help you bring your emotions under Christ's control:

Emotion to Overcome	Principles I Can Use
Lust	2 Timothy 2:22 Titus 2:11-12 1 Peter 4:2
Greed	1 Corinthians 5:5 Ephesians 5:3 1 Peter 5:2
Envy	1 Corinthians 13:4 Galatians 5:25-26 1 Peter 2:1-2

Reread the memory verse. You can learn to be content in every situation because you can do everything through Jesus Christ who gives you the strength to do anything required of you. Let God teach you the secret of spiritual contentment.

 Thank You, Father God, for helping me to conquer the negative influences of lust, greed and envy in my life.

Lord Jesus, teach me how You can fully satisfy the needs of my life.

DAY 6: *Reflections*

In this week's study you have learned how the sins of greed, lust and envy can sneak into your life and send your life out of control. You must turn away from the negative emotions and steer toward God and His Holy Spirit. This will bring you back under God's control.

One way to steer toward God is to read His Word and memorize

Scripture. Yes, that memory thing again. It is important to your growth as a Christian to know His Word for those times you need the right words to help you steer away from temptations. Using Scripture in prayer will also help you stay on the road.

This week's lesson gave you many Scriptures to help you in overcoming the emotional desires that bring havoc into your life. If you haven't already begun making a list of meaningful verses, start now. These are the verses you can use to help you through trying situations.

Through a lifestyle of memorizing Scripture, the Holy Spirit will be able to bring the truths to your mind in difficult times or when temptation comes. When you hide God's Word in your heart, you will truly be storing up treasures in heaven.

Father God, help me to flee from the sin that so easily entangles me; and help me to seek righteousness, godliness, faithfulness, love, endurance and gentleness (see Hebrews 12:1).

Lord God, let me live by the Spirit so that I will not gratify the desires of my sinful nature (see Galatians 5:16).

Holy Father, Your Word says that everything in the world—the cravings of my sinful nature, the lust of my eyes and the boasting of what I have and do—comes, not from You, Father, but from the world and my flesh. You promised that the world and its desires will pass away, but the one who does Your will lives forever. Help me to live in Your will (see 1 John 2:16-17).

DAY 7: Reflections

This week marks the halfway point in your journey through this session. You may have had detours that kept you from following the right route, but you can get back on the highway and continue the journey to success. God doesn't keep account of your detours; He only looks at how you correct your path and come back to Him.

As an adult you have learned how to get to many different places in your city, town or community. You are as familiar with the roads and streets as you are with your own home. Think how full and rich your life would be if you knew the paths of God's Word as well as you do your town or city. Just as there are times when you may get lost in a familiar setting, you can lose your way in life. When lost on the road or in a new part of town, you would pull out a map to find your way back. The Bible is your map for finding your way back on God's road for your life.

The Bible verses you memorize will become the landmarks for seeking God's will and plan in your life. Memorized verses become a beacon of light to guide you to the Father during times of stress, temptation or difficulty. Those verses become prayers that waft toward heaven as incense pleasing to God. He listens, hears and answers.

Lord, Your Word is clear that those who are self-seeking and who reject the truth and follow evil will experience Your wrath and anger (see Romans 2:8).[3]

Father God, continue to teach me. Help me to recognize what is in accordance with the truth that is in Jesus (see Ephesians 4:21).[4]

My faithful God, I thank You for the grace, mercy and peace from You, the Father, and from Jesus Christ, Your Son, that is with me in truth and love (see 2 John 3).[5]

Lord, help me to learn the secret of being content in any and every situation, whether well fed or hungry, whether living in plenty or in want. I can do everything through Him who gives me strength (see Philippians 4:12-13).

Notes

1. W. E. Vine, *Vine's Complete Expository Dictionary of Old and New Testament Words*, ed. Merrill F. Under and William White, Jr. (Nashville, TN: Thomas Nelson, 1996), n.p.
2. Ibid.
3. Beth Moore, *Praying God's Word* (Nashville, TN: Broadman and Holman Publishers, 2000), p. 80.
4. Ibid., p. 81.
5. Ibid., p. 83.

GROUP PRAYER REQUESTS   TODAY'S DATE:_____

NAME	REQUEST	RESULTS

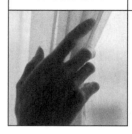

SELF-ESTEEM UNDER CONTROL

MEMORY VERSE

Do not think of yourself more highly than you ought,
but rather think of yourself with sober judgment, in
accordance with the measure of faith God has given you.

Romans 12:3

How should you, as a Christian, feel about yourself? If your self-esteem becomes inflated, you can fall into the sins of pride, arrogance and selfish ambition. If your self-esteem is inadequate, you diminish your value and potential in Christ. The challenge is to think of yourself with "sober judgment, in accordance with the measure of faith God has given you."

In this week's study, you'll learn principles that will help you keep your self-esteem under Christ's control. You'll discover how to develop a clear picture of who you are in Christ. Plus you'll explore how the biblical teachings on humility and greatness impact self-esteem.

DAY 1: *A Renewed Mind and a Clear Picture*

How you see yourself influences how you live, how you interact with others, even how you relate to God. As a Christian, your relationship with Jesus provides the basis for checking your value as a person. In Christ, you can develop healthy and balanced self-esteem that strengthens you and keeps your life under control.

Romans 12:2 warns against conforming to the patterns of this world.

➤ What does the verse tell you to do, instead of conforming?

➤ What patterns do most people use for determining their self-esteem?

Did you think of things the world system values highly and gives high priority? Internalizing the principles of physical beauty, power, possessions or position leads many to assess their own value. They may ask themselves the following questions:

🍎 *Am I beautiful enough?*
🍎 *Have I accumulated the right things?*
🍎 *Am I in a position of influence?*
🍎 *Do I have personal power?*

➤ To what degree have you allowed physical beauty, position, possessions or power to determine your self-esteem?

➤ Which one of these four areas of comparison has most affected your own feeling of self-worth?

➤ Are there other factors that have influenced your self-esteem? Be specific.

As Christians we need our minds to be renewed by God's Word and His Holy Spirit so that we can break free from the world's pattern of assessing value. With a renewed mind, you will learn about the good, pleasing and perfect will of God—the perfect pattern for your life. Romans 12:3-8 focuses on God's plans for your life based on your spiritual gifts. Embedded in these verses is the challenge to think about yourself with "sober judgment."

➻ Summarize Romans 12:3-8 in your own words.

➻ To what degree are you allowing God's biblical truth to determine your self-esteem?

➻ What analogy does James 1:23-25 use to explain the importance of living out what you learn in the Bible?

Romans 12:3 presents you with a great challenge: to evaluate your life with sober judgment. You know the bull's-eye on your target: healthy self-esteem based on an accurate assessment of your life, your strengths and your weaknesses.

 Heavenly Father, use the Bible like a mirror in my life to allow me to see myself as You see me.

Lord God, use Your Word to renew my mind, so I can break out of the patterns that others use to assess my value as a person.

DAY 2: *Inflated Self-Esteem*

If your target is healthy self-esteem, you must guard against overshooting that target and developing an inflated self-esteem instead. One evidence of inflated self-esteem is pride.

➻ According to Proverbs 3:34, how does God respond to proud people?

"Pride" means an overly high opinion of oneself; exaggerated self-esteem. W. E. Vine noted that in the Bible, pride is always used in the negative sense of being arrogant and disdainful.[1]

Another component of inflated self-esteem is an illusion of greatness, which develops into arrogance. In Matthew 20:20-24, the mother of James and John, the disciples, wanted greatness for her sons. She asked Jesus for prominence in His kingdom for them.

➳ How did the other disciples respond to her request? Why do you think they were upset?

➳ First Timothy 6:17 connects arrogance with wealth, implying that as wealth increases, so does arrogance. In your opinion, what is the connection? How can we guard against becoming arrogant?

"Arrogance" means being full of unwarranted pride or self-importance. In the New Testament we read of arrogant people who challenged the apostle Paul's authority and others who were rebellious and not afraid to slander spiritual beings.

➳ According to 1 Corinthians 4:18-21, some in the church at Corinth were challenging Paul's authority. What was his warning to them?

➳ How does 2 Peter 2:10,12 describe spiritual rebels and arrogant men?

⤳ What evidence of inflated self-esteem is found in James 3:14-16? What does such selfishness produce?

The drive to obtain a particular objective—wealth, fame, advancement—can become self-centered. Left unchecked, selfishness can dominate, creating the notion that people are expendable as long as the objective is achieved. Inflated self-esteem leads to those characteristics that set you up to face God's opposition.

Jesus' disciples discussed their relative greatness on a regular basis, arguing over which of them was destined for the top positions in the kingdom to come. In all probability, the disciples were probably most upset because James and John were honing in on the positions they were also coveting.

There is nothing wrong with being great or famous. Billy Graham is a perfect example of a man of widespread fame. He is known throughout the world. However, he never gives glory to himself; the glory always goes to God. No matter what the reason behind your search for greatness, you must be careful that pride and arrogance don't cloud your purpose and lead to an inflated self-esteem.

⤳ Is there evidence of inflated self-esteem in your life?

⤳ Is pride, arrogance or selfish ambition your motivation? If so, how are you going to deal with this problem?

 Heavenly Father, thank You for loving and caring for me. Help me to be the person You want me to be through the power of the Holy Spirit.

Dear Lord, I pray for You to remove the destructive forces of pride, arrogance or selfish ambition from my life.

DAY 3: *Inadequate Self-Esteem*

While it's possible to overshoot the target of healthy self-esteem and develop inflated self-esteem, many people undershoot the target and develop inadequate self-esteem. For a Christian, inflated self-esteem is wrong, but so is inadequate self-esteem. Because of Jesus Christ, people who struggle to find a sense of value have hope.

If you struggle with inadequate self-esteem, remember your incredible value as a person.

> ➣ According to Romans 5:10, what price did God willingly pay for you?

Value is established according to the highest price someone is willing to pay. God established the value for your life when He paid for you with the death of Christ. Jesus died while we were all still rebelling against God, so we didn't earn or deserve Christ's sacrifice. God simply paid the incredible price for each of us, including you.

Inadequate self-esteem leaves you doubting your value, gifts and potential in Christ. Without a healthy sense of self-esteem, you can become self-absorbed, focusing so fully on your own needs that you have no energy left to meet the needs of others. Romans 12:3-8 focuses on the contribution individuals can make as they use the spiritual gifts God gives them. If you struggle with inadequate self-esteem, remember that God has gifted you to make a contribution to His kingdom.

> ➣ Considering Romans 12:3-8, what contribution can you make as part of Christ's Body?

> ➣ Perhaps you have forgotten your spiritual potential; according to Ephesians 3:20, what can God do through you?

Throughout the New Testament Jesus told parables that illustrated the worth He puts on each individual. Consider the story of the shepherd and the lost sheep in Luke 15:4-6.

➣ What does this parable tell you about your worth in the eyes of Jesus?

➣ What does John 10:14-15 tell you about the love of Jesus, the great Shepherd?

If Jesus loves you so much that He is willing to die for you, then you should also see yourself as the redeemed child of God that you are. David gave us an answer for those who don't value their bodies as the handiwork of God but look at themselves as inadequate.

➣ How does Psalm 139:13-16 make you feel about your worth as a person?

As a person, you are valuable because God made you. As a Christian, you are valuable because Christ died for you. You have a contribution to make as part of the Body of Christ because God gifted you. Plus you have unlimited potential because of what Christ can do through you.

 Father God, thank You for making me who I am—a valuable person in Your kingdom.

Heavenly Father, help me to see myself as You see me and value myself as You value me.

DAY 4: An Accurate Map

Driving through a new city can cause confusion without a map. Suppose you are driving through Dallas, Texas. Unknown to you, the map you are using has a major problem. The title says "Dallas," but in reality it is a map of Seattle. The map is well printed, clear and easy to read. Yet no matter how carefully you follow it, you keep getting lost. You call some friends who tell you, "Just try harder" and "All you need is a positive mental attitude." Of course, if your map is wrong, neither hard work nor positive thinking can help. You don't need advice; you need a new map—an accurate map of Dallas!

➺ Romans 12:3 is a description of the map you need for your life; what should characterize this map?

For you to think of yourself more or less highly than you should is inappropriate. Your goal is sober judgment. Seek reality and accuracy as God gives you the ability to do so. Look at yourself and see yourself from His perspective.

If you were to prepare a personal balance sheet on your life, could you do so accurately? Consider the spiritual, emotional, social and physical aspects of your life. What are your assets and liabilities in these four areas?

	Assets	Liabilities
Spiritual		
Emotional		
Social		
Physical		

➤ What does Romans 12:6a tell you about your assets in the eyes of God?

➤ What does Romans 12:6-8 tell you about using your assets?

Every individual has value in the eyes of God. He is the one who gives you your personality and your gifts. He doesn't want you to be ignorant about the spiritual gifts He has given you. Paul explained that true ministry is found in the exercising of spiritual gifts.

➤ What is Paul saying about the different gifts in 1 Corinthians 12:4-6?

God determines what gifts we have or don't have. Why then would we question the Spirit and complain or be depressed because we don't have the same gifts another may have? Just as Paul reminded you not to think too highly of yourself, the Spirit will remind you not to think yourself unworthy or untalented.

God's love is unconditional, and His love is your reason to feel worthy. He will help you view your life with sober judgment in all areas.

 Heavenly Father, I seek Your wisdom in having an accurate understanding of my assets and liabilities.

Dear Lord, help me to view my life with sober judgment and in accordance with the measure of faith You have given me.

DAY 5: *Humility and Self-Esteem*

Charles Spurgeon once said, "Humility is to make a right estimate of one's self." Balanced, healthy self-esteem begins with an accurate personal map of your life. Because of Christ and His work in your life, you can frankly assess the strengths you find, knowing they are gifts from God. Likewise, you can accept your weaknesses, knowing even they can become platforms through which God can demonstrate His strength. With an accurate assessment of life comes humility—we are people who have reason for humility!

God doesn't want you to have low self-esteem, but He also doesn't want you to be filled with pride.

⟐ According to James 4:6, how does God respond to you when you exhibit pride?

⟐ What does He give you when you demonstrate humility?

God loves you because you are His child, not because of the great feats or the successes in your life. Another type of pride is exhibited when one thinks of oneself as better than others.

⟐ According to Matthew 6:1,5, what did Jesus have to say about those who do their works so that others may see their goodness?

⟐ In Matthew 20:26, Jesus explained how to become great. Write His teaching on greatness in your own words.

➤ What example of greatness did Jesus give in Matthew 20:28?

As you develop true self-esteem resulting from your relationship with Jesus, you can shift your focus from yourself to the needs of others. As you serve others in humility, your life will achieve true greatness, following the model Jesus demonstrated.

➤ Romans 8:31 is a rhetorical question. Read the passage and then complete the following statement as the opposite of the question:

If _____ is against us, what does it matter who is

_____ us.

You cannot overcome God's opposition. It's great to think about God being *for you*. But if God is against you, it really doesn't matter who *is* for you. Inflated self-esteem and the pride that accompanies it are lethal in life because pride positions you in opposition to God.

➤ How does John 1:16 describe the grace God gives to the humble?

God will guard you from pride and help you live humbly before Him if you ask. His grace will bring you one blessing after another. Thank God that you will become great in His kingdom as you learn to humbly serve others!

 Thank You, Heavenly Father, for loving me and sending Your grace to give blessings in my life.

Father God, shift my eyes off my own needs and to the needs of people around me.

DAY 6: *Reflections*

In this week's study you have learned what a valuable person you are in God's eyes. He is the only one you need to please. You have been challenged to build your self-esteem on your strengths and to build up your weaknesses with the help of the Holy Spirit. With your focus on the Holy Spirit, you don't have time to develop arrogance, pride and selfish ambition in your life.

Most Christians need occasional reminders to keep their pride and ambition under control. You are probably no different. If you are now in the habit of finding Bible verses to memorize, you will find several that will help you with self-esteem.

Read James 4:6 and Philippians 2:3. Both of these verses are short and to the point, which makes them easy to memorize. Charles Stanley writes, "Humility is quick to confess sin and slow to point it out in others. Humility asks for and receives God's forgiveness and in turn is quick to forgive others. Humility is content to be behind the scenes."2

The book of Proverbs is full of verses that have to do with the characteristics of man. The following all concern pride: Proverbs 8:13; 16:18; 21:4; 26:12 and 27:2. All of these verses warn of the danger of pride and arrogance. This isn't to say that you shouldn't be proud of your accomplishments, but give God the glory for helping you to reach your goals.

The following prayers give you examples to use in writing your own prayers using Scripture:

Heavenly Father, help me to humble myself under Your mighty hand so that I may be exalted in Your time (see 1 Peter 5:6).

Lord God, make me like a tree planted by the rivers of water, that brings forth fruit in season so that whatever I do shall prosper (see Psalm 1:3).

My Holy God, let me do nothing through selfish ambition or conceit, but in lowliness of mind let me esteem others to be better than myself (see Philippians 2:3).

DAY 7: *Reflections*

The goal of the lessons this week is to help you realize the incredible potential you have as a child of God. You have seen Jesus as a role model of service and humility. He is the One on whom your life should focus. God will give you the wisdom you need for making wise choices.

Let's evaluate what you have done so far in First Place. Are you following the commitments you made to First Place? Many members find following each one of them every week to be a difficult task. Concentrate on as many as you can for the upcoming week. Combining commitments is easy with the Bible study, memory verse, Scripture reading and prayer. These fit naturally together. When you attend the meeting, you have completed one more. Usually the most difficult are exercise, keeping the CR and following the Live-It plan. Concentrate on these as you do your daily studies and have prayer time.

Be careful about evaluating your success by the amount of weight lost. A change in attitude and lifestyle and a focus on the Holy Spirit are more valuable than a few pounds lost. Any weight you lose in the program comes as a result of your attitude and willingness to give complete control of your life over to God.

In the following principles set forth this week, write your own brief sentence prayer for each one that you can claim personally. During the remainder of the study, find verses of Scripture that fit the following principles, and use them as a basis for prayer.

- I accept God's assessment of me as a valuable person.
- I have a contribution to make with my life as I use my spiritual gifts.
- In Christ, I have incredible potential.
- I understand my strengths and weaknesses.
- I recognize that I have ample reason for humility.
- I receive God's grace as I live in humility.
- I follow Jesus' model of service and learn His lessons of greatness.

Notes

1. W. E. Vine, *Vine's Complete Expository Dictionary of Old and New Testament Words*, ed. Merrill F. Under and William White, Jr. (Nashville, TN: Thomas Nelson, 1996), n.p.
2. Charles Stanley, *In Touch with God* (Nashville, TN: Thomas Nelson, 1997), p. 109.

GROUP PRAYER REQUESTS TODAY'S DATE:_____

NAME	REQUEST	RESULTS

WORDS UNDER CONTROL

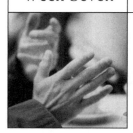

MEMORY VERSE

If anyone considers himself religious and yet does not keep a tight rein on his tongue, he deceives himself and his religion is worthless.

James 1:26

The battle for control of your life is not complete until you fight and win the battle of the tongue!

Words are like tools. In the hands of a trained craftsman, they can create things of beauty and inspiration. However, in careless hands words can harm—even destroy. For that reason, James wrote in his epistle that the impact of our spiritual life can be neutralized if we fail to control our words.

In this week's study, you'll explore what the Bible says about speech. You'll learn about words that hurt and words that heal. You'll also gain insights into the potential for using words for God's glory.

DAY 1: *Words and Their Control*

Compared to controlling your actions, thoughts or emotions, it seems less critical that you control your speech. In reality, the Bible speaks with great force and clarity about the importance of developing tongue-control. Until you can control what comes out of your mouth, you will continue to be vulnerable—a mouth out of control can lead to a life out of control.

Throughout the book of Proverbs, there are great words of wisdom about controlling one's tongue. When deciding what to say, remaining silent at times might be the wiser action.

The following verses explain some of the benefits of controlling the tongue. Read each verse; then write the benefits beside each.

≫ Proverbs 10:19

≫ Proverbs 17:28

≫ Proverbs 21:23

≫ 1 Peter 3:10

Remember Thumper in the classic movie *Bambi?* He quoted his father's advice: "If you can't say somethin' nice, don't say nothin' at all." The first step in developing self-control is to simply say nothing.

≫ In the memory verse for this week, James had strong words for people who couldn't control their tongues. In what sense do such people deceive themselves?

As God begins to work in your life, one of the first things He wants to transform is your speech. James 1:26 implies that people who call themselves Christians, yet cannot control their tongues, are living in a spiritual fantasy. If God is really at work in their hearts, their speech will demonstrate His controlling influence. Religious words alone, without the Holy Spirit's presence within, are worthless.

Heavenly Father, help me to know when to be silent and when to speak in Your name.

Dear Lord, help me to be careful about my speech so that my words will bring honor to You.

DAY 2: Words and Their Potential

Just as sparks from a campfire can ignite a forest fire, so our words can ravage the lives of others. Since words express thoughts and ideas, our speech serves as a barometer of the spiritual pressure level of our hearts. The potential of words can build up others with praise or hurt them with anger, bitterness or thoughtlessness.

Thoughts become kindling for emotions. Once emotions blaze and begin to burn out of control, actions easily spin out of control as well. Spoken words tend to reinforce thoughts. If we control our thought life, we will better control our tongue.

➥ In James 3:3-8, what are the analogies given for the power of the tongue and how does each relate to the negative impact of the tongue?

➥ How can each of these analogies relate to the positive impact of our words?

➥ What is the warning found in verse 8?

In direct opposition to the dangerous aspects of words is the great spiritual potential of kind words. The spiritual potential of words is the most important reason for bringing our words under control. It is incredible that God uses everyday people to communicate His truth.

➥ Paul said his words were effective because of God's power. After reading 1 Corinthians 2:4-5 and 1 Thessalonians 1:5, describe an experience you have had when the Holy Spirit gave you special words while you were speaking to someone about Christ.

➳ According to 1 Corinthians 2:13, what is the source of our witness to others?

➳ How have you been sharing what you have learned in the First Place program?

How would you rate yourself on the "Tongue Control Scale"? Check the box beside those statements that best describe your progress in tongue control.

☐ I remain silent when I should. God has helped me know when to speak.

☐ Most times, I know when to stop talking. I'm not perfect but improving.

☐ Half the time I know what to say or when to stop talking; other times I get myself into trouble or hurt others.

☐ It's a struggle for me to control my talking. I feel a need to express my opinion.

☐ People love to hear me talk; I always know the right thing to say.

➳ What is the implication of Matthew 12:34-37 for a Christian?

God has given you the means by which you can tell others about Him. In the same manner, the very same means can undo all your hard work. Pray as David did in Psalm 141:3: "Set a guard over my mouth, O LORD; keep watch over the door of my lips."

Lord, help me to learn the discipline of keeping silent in order to listen to others and to learn to use words that will bring comfort.

Heavenly Father, thank You for the privilege of telling others about Your love and mercy. Help me to use my words to honor You and build up others.

DAY 3: *Words That Stir Up Trouble and Hurt People*

The Bible warns against many types of character qualities and behaviors that are inappropriate or harmful: Quarreling, lying and flattery for gain are only three examples. These three ways of interacting with people are all ways we can use words—words that stir up trouble.

In addition to stirring up trouble, words have the ability to hurt or shut people out. French philosopher Blaise Pascal[1] once said:

> Cold words freeze people, and hot words scorch them, and bitter words make them bitter, and wrathful words make them wrathful. Kind words also produce their image on men's souls; and a beautiful image it is. They soothe, and quiet, and comfort the hearer.

➤ How does Proverbs 12:18 impact you?

Two types of negative speech, slander and gossip, also make deep cuts. Read the following verses; then write what each passage says about the seriousness of slander and gossip:

➤ Ephesians 4:31

✎ Romans 1:29-30

When you quarrel, you lose your focus on truth, and emotions drive discussions. When you lie, you leave the truth all together. When you flatter, you use truths and half-truths to manipulate and influence. All three types of words plant seeds of discord in your relationships, which ultimately produces trouble! Read the following verses; then write a summary of the insights you gain:

✎ Romans 16:17-18

✎ Colossians 3:8-9

✎ James 4:1-2

✎ Have you ever been the victim of gossip or slander? How did you feel?

Pray that you will never forget the pain those words caused you and that you will always use words with caution as you deal with others.

 Heavenly Father, help me to speak the truth in love as I deal with people.

Father God, help me to always speak words of love and comfort—words that will make peace, not trouble.

DAY 4: *Words That Build Your Relationship with God*

Our first goal should be to know when to keep silent and when to speak. The second is to rid our speech of words that stir up trouble or hurt people. Our third challenge is to build relationships with our words. Throughout the psalms, David and others used words to exalt, praise, thank and worship God, as well as to confess sin to God.

The following are examples of using words that worship, praise, exalt and thank the Lord, and one verse is about confession of sin. After reading the verses, choose the word that best describes the theme of each one.

_____	Psalm 18:49	a.	Worship
_____	Psalm 30:12	b.	Praise
_____	Psalm 32:5	c.	Exaltation
_____	Psalm 34:3	d.	Thanks
_____	Psalm 100:2	e.	Confession

When your words are pleasing to God, you will not hurt others, embarrass yourself or bring dishonor to the name of God. Let your words be based on those of David in Psalm 19:14.

➽ Write your own prayer based on Psalm 19:14.

 Heavenly Father, may my words always be in praise and honor of Your holy name.

Holy God, I give thanks to You for the many blessings You bestow on me and for sending Your Son to forgive my sins, so I may have eternal life.

DAY 5: *Words That Build Relationships with People*

Not only can your words build your relationship with God, but they can also become tools for building your relationships with people.

➤ What are the opposites described in Proverbs 15:4?

Just as Jesus' words brought healing to the bodies and souls of His followers, so should your words be those of healing relationships with others. The verses below all refer to words that build relationships. Read each passage; then write the words from each that will help to build relationships.

➤ Words that express gratitude: Ephesians 1:15-16

➤ Words that bring people together: Colossians 3:13

➤ Words that guide others in the right direction: Colossians 3:16

➤ Words that give hope: 1 Thessalonians 5:11,14

➤ Words that build up: 1 Peter 2:17

Think of the people with whom you speak each week and recall your most recent conversations. Circle the words above that could be used to describe your conversations. If you discover that you are using negative words as you interact with people, confess that to God and He will guide you into using encouraging and healing words.

➤ Read/recite the memory verse from week 3—Philippians 4:8. List the words from this verse that you are reminded to think on.

Heavenly Father, help me to limit my words to those that will build my relationships with people.

DAY 6: *Reflections*

In this week's study we focused on the importance of words in our relationships with others and with God. We know that words can tear down as well as build up. They can heal or cause great pain. They can comfort or bring great sorrow. Words are our primary means of communication with others. Whether those words are written or spoken, they convey our thoughts, ideas, plans, hopes and attitudes.

God has given you the opportunity to experience His power in your life when you speak. You don't have to be a preacher or an evangelist. When you use what you have learned in the Bible and simply tell others about it, God has promised to bless what you say and how you use His Word in the lives of others.

Many opportunities arise in your daily walk when particular Scriptures may help in conveying ideas to others. The Word of God is true and is an infallible source in helping you to convey the power of God and His love to those who don't know Him.

Along with memorizing verses to use in your prayer time, seek out verses that will help you in witnessing to others. These can be words of sympathy, understanding, conviction, praise, thanks or love. You have heard the phrase "What would Jesus do?" Consider also the phrase "What would Jesus say?" Too many times Christians speak before thinking, but if you carefully consider your words as you do your actions, your words will more likely be those God would have you say.

God has given you the privilege of telling others about Him. If you seek Him, He will help you use words to honor Him.

➤ In Proverbs 15:1-2,4, you will notice that the contrasts in these verses show the difference between righteousness and wickedness. What is the implication for you as you build relationships with others?

The following prayers concern speaking to others:

Heavenly Father, let my words always be pleasant, a honeycomb sweet to the soul and healing to the bones (see Proverbs 16:24).

O Lord, put a guard over my mouth and tongue to keep me from disaster; keep watch over the door of my lips (see Psalm 141:3).

Let the words of my mouth and the meditations of my heart be pleasing in Your sight, O Lord, my Rock and my Redeemer (see Psalm 19:14).

DAY 7: *Reflections*

Another focus of the Bible study this week was to praise, exalt, worship and thank God for all He has done for you. You also learned how the Word of God can be used to teach, instruct, forgive, challenge, inspire, edify, affirm, honor, pardon and encourage others.

How have you used words this week to edify, encourage, inspire or challenge others? One of the commitments of First Place is encouragement. A word of encouragement to a fellow class member, either written or spoken, may be just the thing that member needs to keep on and not give up.

Each week, as you memorize the verse, find a way to use it to speak to someone about what God has done for you or what God can do for them.

In addition, use Scripture to give God praise and thanks for what He can do and has done.

If you are experiencing problems in memorizing Scripture, find ways to use that verse every day. Make it personal for you. E-mail is another good way to communicate with others, and you can always sign off with the memory verse or another verse that is important to you. At work, stop, take a moment and write down the verse on a piece of paper without looking at it first. At home, stop and say as much of the verse as you can without looking it up. You will find it easier and easier to write or repeat each time you do.

The Scripture memory book and the CD of the memory verses are additional helps to aid your memorization. Because God's Word is always true, praying God's Word means you are praying the truth. What better way is there to communicate with God?

Instead of written prayers as examples this week, you are going to use Scriptures to write your own prayers to God.

➤ Praise—Use words to express gratitude for who God is: Psalm 9:1-2

➤ Worship—Use words to express your love: Psalm 95:6-7

➤ Thanksgiving—Use words to express gratitude for what God has done for you: Psalm 118:29

➤ Write a prayer using this week's memory verse.

Note
1. Blaise Pascal (1623-1662).

GROUP PRAYER REQUESTS   TODAY'S DATE:_____

NAME	REQUEST	RESULTS

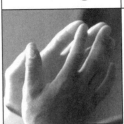
SPIRITUAL DISCIPLINES HELP

MEMORY VERSE

*If anyone would come after me, he must deny himself
and take up his cross daily and follow me.*

Luke 9:23

There are basic disciplines that are essential for spiritual growth. Much has been written about this topic, using various models to help people remember the disciplines. Although the presentations and priorities vary on the fundamental elements recommended, there is virtual consensus.

In this week's study, we'll focus on the discipline of the Cross. In the process, we'll learn more about spiritual disciplines and the role they play in keeping our lives under Christ's control.

DAY 1: *Make Three Basic Commitments*

As disciples of Jesus Christ, we should desire to please Him. As our Lord, Jesus deserves to control and direct our lives. With Him empowering us, we can avoid many of the negative situations that develop when life slips out of control. Our motivation, however, should not simply be to avoid problems. We should seek to live Christ-controlled lives for higher reasons. First, with your life under control, you can use your energy in positive ways, rather than dealing with the negative consequences that always accompany sin. Second, as you live a Christ-controlled life, all that you do becomes a testimony of the difference Christ makes in everyday people.

In Luke 9:23, Jesus lays out three basic commitments that are a part of discipleship.

≫ What are those three commitments?

1.

2.

3.

≫ What evidence in your life right now indicates that you have made any or all of these basic commitments?

As with many areas of Christian life, you might think, *But how do I do this? How do these grand-sounding commitments translate into practical steps I can take each day?*

If you wanted to act on these three commitments more completely, what would you do? In the spaces below, write some steps that might be appropriate.

≫ How would you deny yourself?

≫ How would you take up your cross?

≫ How would you follow Jesus?

As you study this week, think of how Luke 9:23 applies to your commitments to the First Place program.

Father God, help me to use the study this week to learn practical ways to deny myself, take up my cross and follow after You as Your disciple.

Lord God, help me and guide me as I work toward the commitments I made to the First Place program.

DAY 2: *Abide in Christ and Live in His Word*

The first commitment Jesus calls you to make is to deny yourself. How strange His challenge sounds in a world absorbed with self! Some say Jesus' command illustrates how Christianity undermines healthy self-esteem. "How can you feel good about yourself and deny yourself at the same time?" is the argument. Of course, the critics forget that Jesus commanded Christians to love their neighbors as they love themselves. You cannot fulfill that commandment without a healthy sense of self-love! No, when Jesus calls you to deny yourself, He expects you to renounce self-centered living and replace it with Christ-centered being.

In John 15:5, Jesus explained the relationship His disciples were to maintain with Him.

➤ On the basis of the analogy He used, what insights can you gain into your own relationship with Jesus?

➤ Jesus remains in you through His Holy Spirit. How do you remain in Him?

➤ What did Jesus mean by the phrase "apart from me, you can do nothing"?

It's not enough to deny yourself, take up your cross and place Christ at the center of your life, abiding in Him. What else do you need? You must add basic spiritual disciplines to your life. One of these is *living in the Word*. By studying the Bible, you strengthen Christ's control in your life.

➤ Considering John 8:31-32, how does what Jesus said apply to your own life?

➤ Jesus said His truth will set you free; have you experienced that freedom in your life? If so, give a specific example.

Jesus called you to live a Christ-focused life, rather than one that is self-focused. He called you to live a Christ-dependent life, instead of living independently. Jesus called you to live in such a way that He can live and work through you. The first basic discipline is to spend time daily with God in His Word. Some call this time their quiet time; others may call it personal devotions. No matter what name you give it, you must spend daily time reading God's Word, praying and seeking His direction.

Have you developed this discipline in your life?

➤ How did you begin this habit?

➤ When do you have your quiet time?

≫ What benefits do you receive?

Spending personal time with God each day is the first basic spiritual discipline of the Christian life. You need to know God's Word before you can live in it. He will empower you and give you the desire to read, study, memorize, understand and apply His Word.

Heavenly Father, strengthen the time I spend with You each day and help me hide Your Word in my heart through the Scriptures I memorize.

Lord God, help me to use Your Word to direct and control my life. Thank You for setting me free through the truth of Your Word.

DAY 3: *Pray in Faith*

The second basic spiritual discipline, according to the memory verse, is to take up your cross. When you pray in faith, you open your life to Christ's control. To find insights into the discipline of prayer, consider John 15:7.

≫ What is the incredible promise in John 15:7 regarding prayer?

≫ What are the two conditions Jesus gives for this promise?

   1.

   2.

➤ What is the promise and the condition for answered prayer found in both Matthew 21:22 and Mark 11:24?

➤ Why do you think Jesus put this condition on our prayers?

You remain in Jesus as you daily spend time with Him in your personal quiet time. You allow His words to remain in you as you read, study, memorize and apply the Bible. Each week as you memorize the verse for the week, you are putting His words in your heart.

Then you must have faith and believe that God will answer you. As stated in Mark 11:24: "Whatever you ask for in prayer, believe that you have received it." God's answers sometimes don't coincide with how or what you want, but God's answer is always the right answer and the one you need.

At the end of each week, on the reflection day, you have been learning the importance of memorizing Scripture and praying God's Word. When you know what the Bible says about prayer and believing God, you will gain confidence in the promise found in 1 John 5:14-15.

➤ What is the promise in which you can have confidence?

➤ How do your personal quiet time and your personal commitment to know and obey the Bible impact the way you pray?

God will help you know Him better as you spend time with Him daily in your quiet time and as you learn more about the Bible. Remember that the Bible is true and the Bible is God's Word. God is truth, and His truth will set you free from the stronghold of whatever keeps you from giving God control of your life.

 Heavenly Father, give me the discipline to read, study and memorize Your Word and to use that Word to direct and control my life.

Father God, help me to know Your perfect will as I read the Bible and pray with confidence in accordance with that will.

DAY 4: *Have Fellowship with Believers*

As we seek to take up our crosses, we will need to add another practical spiritual discipline to our lives: fellowship with believers. Living for Christ in a secular world is a demanding experience. We need the support of other Christians to make it. We also have the opportunity to express Christ's love to fellow believers just as He commanded.

➢ In John 13:34-35, Jesus commanded us to love others. Is it possible to simply decide to love others? How can we do as Jesus commanded and love others—even the difficult people?

➢ What do you learn about love with Jesus as the standard?

Jesus said the identifying mark of His disciples would be love—not high-powered quiet times, not great knowledge of the Bible, not even incredible prayer lives, but love. "Love" is one of the most often used words in the Bible. Look at any concordance and you will find several pages on the words "love," "loving" and "loved." Christ placed such great importance on this aspect of our relationship with both Him and others that it was to be the hallmark of His followers. He demonstrated the greatest love of all when He willingly gave His life to redeem us from sin. We may strive to be like Him, but if we don't have love, we will never reach the goal of being a true disciple.

➤ Think about the time you have spent with your First Place group. What have you learned in this group about the importance of giving love?

➤ What have you learned about receiving love?

➤ Give a few examples of how love is shown within your group.

Christian fellowship is a great privilege. As you spend time with others, you share the life you have in Christ and the love He has given you. God never intended for you to live as a lone-ranger Christian. You must discipline yourself to share your life with others. They need you and you need them.

As you fellowship with believers, you can help others grow spiritually and encourage Christians; consider 2 Corinthians 1:3-4 and 1 Thessalonians 5:11.

Check the box below which best describes your life right now:

☐ I'm excited about what God is doing in my life. I'm ready for Him to do more.

☐ I'm making progress. God is doing more with me now than ever before.

☐ I'm not sure God can do much through my life. Is there hope for change?

God wants you to put your life under His control. He can use you to accomplish His purposes in the world. It's never too late to get started.

 Heavenly Father, thank You for my First Place group and the love they have shown to me.

O Lord, teach me how to give love more abundantly to those in my life and teach me to receive love as I fellowship with them.

DAY 5: *Witness to the World*

Maintaining our role as a witness for Christ is a key discipline in spiritual growth. Not everyone is a great evangelist, but everyone can be a witness. In that role, our responsibility is to give testimony about what Christ has done in our lives.

➥ What is the promise in Acts 1:8?

John 15:5 compares your relationship to Jesus as a branch connected to a vine. Read to see how that analogy is carried a step further.

➥ According to John 15:8, who will receive glory?

➥ What is the fruit you will produce?

➥ What will others know about you from your fruit?

As Jesus works in your life, your life produces spiritual fruit. Jesus works in you, directing and controlling your actions. He accomplishes spiritual work through your life. Part of His work in you will be seen in the fruit of the Spirit listed in Galatians 5:22-23. Read the list again to refresh your memory. The other part of His work in your life is your witness to others.

➤ In Matthew 4:19, what did Jesus mean by "fishers of men"?

➤ How does that statement apply to your life?

➤ How can you show love for your neighbor, a stranger walking down the street, a coworker or someone who has hurt you?

Another aspect of witnessing and loving others is the willingness to go to great lengths to bring a person to the knowledge of Jesus. Jesus went so far as to lay down His life.

➤ Consider John 15:13. How can you lay down your life for others?

God has called you to a life of ministry—meeting needs. Your First Place commitments and spiritual disciplines give you resources to meet needs in other people's lives. As you live in God's Word, you can teach others what you are learning. As you pray in faith, you can focus on others' needs through intercessory prayer. As you witness to the world, you will introduce others to your Savior.

Holy God, help me to live as Your disciple under Your control, bearing spiritual fruit and bringing You glory.

Heavenly Father, give me opportunities to be a witness for You this week and to have the privilege of helping another person discover Your love.

DAY 6: *Reflections*

This week's study focused on the spiritual disciplines that help you follow Christ. You learned about the promises that when you pray believing in His name, He will answer. When those prayers contain the Scripture verses you memorize, God is pleased. The words are sweet incense as they make their way to heaven.

Several verses from this week's study make excellent Scriptures to memorize. Matthew 21:22; Mark 11:24; Luke 9:23; John 15:7 and Acts 1:8 are verses that hold great promise for a Christian. These are verses you can count on in times of need or stress or to remind you how the Holy Spirit empowers you when your life is in His control. When you hold verses like these in your heart, any stronghold that threatens to overtake your life will be defeated by the Holy Spirit.

Heavenly Father, I count it joy when I fall into various trials, for I know that the testing of my faith produces patience. Let patience have its perfect work so that I may be perfect and complete, lacking nothing (see James 1:2-4).

O Lord, grant me patience, for You have said to wait on You and be strong and take heart (see Psalm 27:14).

Lord God, I trust in You forever, for You, my Lord, are the Rock eternal (see Isaiah 26:4).

DAY 7: *Reflections*

As you center your life on the three commitments of this week's memory verse, you allow Christ's control of your life. As you maintain your relationship with God through your quiet time, you deny yourself—setting aside a self-focused life—and abide in Christ instead. You take up your cross daily as you maintain the four basic spiritual disciplines of living in the Word, praying in faith, fellowshiping with believers and witnessing to the world. The final commitment of following Christ flows naturally from the other two commitments. As you follow Christ, He can work in your life to touch others in ministry.

Being able to minister to those in need is another excellent reason for memorizing Scripture. One strategy you might use is to categorize the verses you memorize. They may be broken down into categories such as promises for times of need, handling fear, power of the Holy Spirit, prayer, knowing God's love, resisting temptation, the plan of salvation, God's will or any category that speaks to your own personal needs.

When you have Scripture memorized, you will have a source of strength and power that is available only to those who believe in Jesus Christ, abide in Him, trust His Word, pray in His name and live in obedience to His commands. Take these powerful weapons and use them to minister to others. The more involved you are with God's Word in reading, studying, praying and ministering to others, the stronger your weapons become when you are faced with temptation or trials.

Keeping the commitments of First Place is easier for a life under God's control. This does not mean that you will keep them faithfully every day, every week no matter what. Most members find themselves lacking in one or two areas at one time or another. You have tapes, Scripture memory and reading, Bible study, a class roster, a commitment record and loving leaders and group members available to help you with the nine commitments. You are not in this alone. Not only is God beside you for encouragement and support, but you also have your group members and leader(s) who are ready to pray for you and encourage you. If you seek His face, He will give you the time you need to study the Bible and pray, and He will help to make memorizing Scripture easier for you.

As for You, my God, Your way is perfect; Your Word is flawless. You are my shield and I take refuge in You (see Psalm 18:30).

Thank You, God, that You know Your sheep. You have given me eternal life and I shall never perish. No one can snatch me out of Your hand (see John 10:27-29).

Father God, I thank You that because I am in Christ, Satan, the prince of this world, has no hold on me (see John 14:30).

Holy Lord, help me to deny myself, take up my cross and follow You daily (see Luke 9:23).

GROUP PRAYER REQUESTS   TODAY'S DATE:_____

NAME	REQUEST	RESULTS

FRIENDS CAN HELP

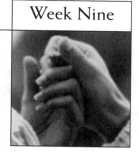

MEMORY VERSE

Let us consider how we may spur one another
on toward love and good deeds. Let us not give up
meeting together, as some are in the habit of doing,
but let us encourage one another—all the more
as you see the Day approaching.

Hebrews 10:24-25

Paul Tournier once said, "There are two things we cannot do alone: one is be married and the other is to be a Christian." Far too many Christians try to keep their lives under spiritual control without the support of other believers. The Christian life is not experienced solo. God designed Christians to be interdependent, bound together through their relationship with Jesus Christ.

In this week's study, we'll learn more about the positive impact other Christians can have on our lives. We'll discover how God uses other people to encourage our spiritual development. Never did God intend for you to live the Christian life alone. You need people; people need you.

DAY 1: *Sharing Lives in Truth and Openness*

As the world becomes more crowded and the pace of life accelerates, we've become used to being surrounded by people. Yet while most people are constantly surrounded by people, they are seldom truly with people—connecting with one another. We long to be accepted and loved by others. Personal relationships are essential to healthy spiritual development. Without a network of love and support, our lives can easily slip out of control.

In 1 Thessalonians 2:6-9, Paul described the relationship he developed with a group of Christians.

➤ If you allowed the image of the gentle mother to guide your interaction with other Christians, what changes would you have to make?

➤ Have you ever been in Christian groups where people shared biblical truths without sharing their lives? What did you feel as you participated in that group?

Sometimes, in our excitement to gain knowledge, we might bypass the opportunity to develop relationships. Paul found the proper balance with his Christian friends. He shared God's truth with them, but he also shared his life with them and he grew to love them. When God's truth is shared with love, the potential for growth is incredible.

In addition to sharing your life and God's truths, you must be open with your Christian friends. In order for your friends to be prayer warriors for you, they must know what your needs are. Certainly you can ask for prayer for unnamed requests, but needs shared openly are needs that will be presented to God by Christian friends.

As a Christian, you have the privilege of going directly to God to confess your sins and find cleansing and forgiveness. However, the truth of James 5:16 speaks of the spiritual benefit of your relationships with others, sometime even confessing your sins to them.

➤ What is your initial response to the verse in James?

You need comfort from someone when you hurt. You also need someone to urge you on to live a life worthy of your high calling of God in Christ Jesus. We all need spiritual mothers or fathers who will nurture us. Unfortunately, many Christians never find such a loving group. In 1 Thessalonians 2:11-12, Paul described his role as a spiritual father with Christian friends.

➤ What three things did Paul say he did with his friends?

1.

2.

3.

➤ Have you ever been part of a group in which a spiritual father or mother or the group itself responded to you as Paul did with his friends? Describe the time.

Sharing your needs, shortcomings, love, encouragement, sympathy and testimony with others gives you a supporting foundation that only Christians can truly understand. However, great damage has been done by people misusing the principles in James 5:16. Just because some might misuse this verse, you should not completely reject it. God placed it in the Bible for our benefit. If you have difficulty sharing with a group, you might find a close friend with whom you feel comfortable and ask him or her to be your prayer partner.

In most cases, sensitive issues should be shared in a private setting with a person trained and equipped to help deal with such problems. However, for less personal and intense problems, great good can come as you share honestly with a group of fellow strugglers. Perhaps one way to apply the verse in James is to say to others who share hurts and failures, "God has forgiven you, God loves you, and so do we!"

 Thank You, Lord, for the love and acceptance of Christian friends through whom I can experience Your unconditional love.

Heavenly Father, help me to become a loving and supportive member of my First Place group.

DAY 2: A Place to Find Courage

The pressure of life can drain away our courage. Like Joshua in the Old Testament, we constantly need to hear the words "Be strong and courageous. Do not be [afraid or] terrified" (Joshua 1:9). Discouragement leaves you vulnerable to sin. When you feel there is no reason to keep trying, opportunities to move in negative directions abound. We need regular infusions of encouragement to simply face life.

One reason the First Place program helps people overcome spiritual, weight or other physical problems is the effectiveness of the group meetings. Encouragement is a major component of helping us stay on track with our goals. The nine commitments are essential to the success of the program. Keeping your life under control, especially while working to change lifestyle habits, requires constant support and accountability from Christian friends. The good news is that you *can* change; success is possible—with God's help and a little help from your friends.

In 2 Timothy 4:2, Paul gave Timothy instruction for becoming a more effective minister to his flock.

➣ How can the last part of this verse especially apply to you as a member of First Place?

➣ According to 1 Thessalonians 2:11-12, what three things did Paul do that you can do as a member of First Place to help others?

1.

2.

3.

➤ According to Hebrews 3:13, why is it important to encourage one another?

Encouragement is one of the greatest gifts Christians can give each other. The verses in the following chart will give you insights into your opportunity to give and receive encouragement. Read each verse; then complete the missing phrase.

Scriptures	The Privilege of Encouragement
Romans 1:12	Your spiritual _____ should naturally encourage each other.
Romans 15:4	God uses the _____ to encourage you.
Romans 15:5	God Himself _____ you.
1 Thessalonians 4:18	Encourage each other by Christ's _____ coming.
1 Thessalonians 5:11	Encourage and _____ each other up.
1 Thessalonians 5:14	Encourage the _____ and help the weak.
Titus 1:9	Encourage others with _____ doctrine.
Hebrews 3:13	Encourage one another every _____, all through the day.
Hebrews 10:25	Encourage one another as you _____ together.

God will encourage you as you encourage others.

Lord God, give me the opportunity today to encourage others.

Thank You, Lord, for giving me Christian friends who are supporting me in the First Place program; use me to help others in reaching their goals.

DAY 3: *Help with Those Blind Spots*

One of the main reasons we need the support of Christian friends is that we all have blind spots. There are areas of life, spiritually and emotionally, that you simply may not see clearly. For a variety of reasons, your perspective is distorted. What you perceive to be reality is simply not accurate. In the same way that driving with an inaccurate map creates problems, so living with blind spots complicates life.

Paul warned believers to be careful of judging others and not examining one's own actions.

➤ In Galatians 6:2-5, what instructions did Paul give the Galatians?

➤ How can you apply this to your own blind spots?

➤ In Matthew 7:1-5, Jesus Himself addressed the problem of blind spots. Have you ever judged others, only to discover later that what you saw so clearly in their lives was in your own life, but you hadn't realized it? What did you learn from the situation?

➤ Why do you think it is so easy to see the specks in other people's eyes but overlook the plank in your own eye?

➤ Once you have taken the time to remove the plank from your own eye, how does that prepare you to help with the speck in another person's eye?

Judging others before you look at yourself may cause you to be over-confident in your own life. Test your own actions first and confess your sin; then go to your brother or sister and speak to him or her in love and forgiveness. Removing specks from your eyes is painful enough—much less removing planks. When a group of Christian friends love each other enough to gently deal with one another's blind spots, great spiritual growth can occur. One of the great gifts you can give each other is clear spiritual vision.

 Father God, reveal my blind spots to me, no matter how painful the process may be.

Heavenly Father, give me the opportunity to help others gently remove things from their lives that are hindering their spiritual potential.

DAY 4: *Moving Forward Once Again*

Howard Hendricks defined a fanatic as someone who redoubles his effort once he has lost his way. As a Christian, you may occasionally get stuck in a spiritual loop. Like the nation of Israel did in the desert, you wander in meandering circles going no place in particular. Because of this tendency to lose direction or motivation, God expects you to connect with other Christians who will help you get moving in the right direction once again.

Read the memory verse, Hebrews 10:24-25, again.

➤ In practical terms, what are we to help others do?

Without ongoing support, we may stagnate in our Christian life. Rather than growing in love and living the principles of our faith, we become comfortable. We need Christian friends who love us enough to say "Isn't it about time you got moving again?"

In your own life, there may have been times when you've needed encouragement because you felt like you were treading water or running in place. Your spiritual life seemed to be going nowhere, or you just couldn't motivate yourself to do what you needed to do. Many times a friend or someone close to you will notice discouragement in your life and say or do the thing you most need to hear or do in your life to get you going again.

➤ Think about such a time in your life. Who helped you? What did that person say or do that helped you get back on the right track?

God is faithful and knows when you need help. He will touch you in such a way that you will be aware when someone in your group in First Place or your circle of friends needs a word of encouragement and motivation from you.

In the memory verse, the word "consider" suggests that you need to think about the process you will use to "spur" different people in their spiritual progress. Appropriate words or actions for one person could damage another. As God directs you, your goal should be to do what accomplishes the goal of encouraging your friend in such a way as to move him or her toward increased love and good works. You must consider where people are in their spiritual development.

What sort of action would you use to "spur," or encourage, spiritual growth in the following:

➤ A new Christian?

➤ A mature Christian with a blind spot?

➤ A Christian older than you?

➤ A discouraged Christian?

When you seek God's guidance and pray for your friends, He will give you the right words, the right verse, the right action for each individual.

 Heavenly Father, bring people into my life who will encourage me in my spiritual walk.

Dear Lord, use me to help other Christians to live in love and do good work for Christ.

DAY 5: *Help Through Prayer*

The apostle Paul was one of the most dynamic and effective Christians who ever lived. During his life, he impacted thousands of people, and the repercussions of his life are still being felt today. Paul was a strong, focused, intense Christian. Yet he was a Christian who understood His weaknesses. He depended on his friends. He constantly wrote his friends, asking them, even pleading with them, to pray for him. The pattern in Paul's life of requesting prayer is another way we can keep our spiritual lives under control.

James 5:16 is one example of Paul requesting the prayers of others. In the following chart, you will find many times where Paul requested prayer for specific needs in his life. After reading the verses, complete the missing phrases.

Scriptures	Asking Others to Pray for You
Romans 15:30	Join me in my _____ by praying for me.
Romans 15:31	Pray I will be _____ and my service will be acceptable.
2 Corinthians 1:11	You _____ me when you pray for me.
Ephesians 6:19	Pray that I will _____ make the gospel known.
Colossians 4:3	Pray that God may open the _____ for our gospel message.
Colossians 4:4	Pray that I may proclaim _____ clearly, as I should.
2 Thessalonians 3:1	Pray that the message of the Lord may _____ rapidly.
Philemon 22	I hope to be _____ in answer to your prayers.

When people pray for you and your needs, you allow the Holy Spirit to work in many lives as He ministers to you. The lives of those who pray for you are enriched by connecting with the Lord. God never leaves you alone, and He provides Christian friends to give earthly support to His heavenly ministry.

Thank You, Lord, for sending people into my life who care about me and pray for me.

Father God, help me to become a person who shows love and care for others by becoming a prayer warrior on their behalf.

DAY 6: *Reflections*

Being in a First Place group gives you the perfect opportunity to put into practice the principles studied this week. Your Christian friends give you support and love in times of need. You return that love and support when you pray for a friend, visit or take food when they are ill, or just sit and listen.

One way to minister to your friends is through the Scripture you memorize. Grouping the memory verses into categories that apply to different situations will provide appropriate verses to use in ministry to others. Even if you are not a gifted speaker, sincere words spoken in love give comfort and encouragement to those who need it.

If you haven't already started a notebook, file or a prayer journal for memory verses in addition to the ones in First Place, it isn't too late. Any time is a good time to begin memorizing Scripture, and you will discover what a difference those verses can make in your life and ministry.

The following are verses to use in encouraging someone who is facing difficult times:

O God, You have promised perfect peace to him whose mind is steadfast because he trusts in You. Father, grant that peace to your servant (see Isaiah 26:3).

Father God, my sacrifice to You is a broken spirit, for You have said a broken and contrite heart You will not despise (see Psalm 51:17).

Heavenly Father, thank You for giving me peace. Because I have been justified through faith, I have peace with You through my Lord Jesus Christ (see Romans 5:1).

DAY 7: *Reflections*

Someone once asked Charles Stanley if a person can live by faith and still set goals. He told the person he'd have to think about that. Stanley came to the conclusion that, yes, a person can live by faith and still set goals, but he or she must be sure the goals are God's goals for his or her life.[1]

When you set goals for yourself, where do you go for guidance? David said, "Your word is a lamp to my feet and a light for my path" (Psalm 119:105). Go to the Bible for guidance. Hide God's Word in your heart and you will always have His light to direct your decisions and actions throughout your day.

Think about the decisions you have made in your life. How has God played a part in those decisions? Sometimes you may make a decision you think God wants you to make and then discover that God wants you to go an entirely different way. Knowing God's Word and using it in all situations gives you access to the power you have as a child of His.

If you are still having difficulty memorizing Scripture, ask a group member or your First Place leader to help you. They will be able to give you suggestions and listen as you repeat the verse. If you are more of a visual learner, write the verse several times until you can easily write it down without looking at it. However you memorize a verse, it will become a valuable weapon in your battle against Satan and overcoming any obstacle that stands in the way of walking closer with Him.

> Lord, please help me listen to advice and accept instruction so that in the end I will be wise (see Proverbs 19:20).[2]
>
> Lord, no matter what kind of suffering my addictions have caused me, I thank You that my present sufferings are not worth comparing with the glory that will be revealed in me (see Romans 8:18).[3]
>
> Dear God, no matter what I once was, I have been washed, I have been sanctified, and I have been justified in the name of the Lord Jesus Christ and by the Spirit of our God (see 1 Corinthians 6:11).[4]
>
> Heavenly Father, help me consider how I can spur others toward love and good deeds. Don't allow me to give up meeting with other Christians, but let me encourage others (see Hebrews 10:24-25).

Notes
1. Charles Stanley, *In Touch with God* (Nashville, TN: Thomas Nelson, 1997), p. 135.
2. Beth Moore, *Praying God's Word* (Nashville, TN: Broadman and Holman Publishers, 2000), p. 132.
3. Ibid., p.136.
4. Ibid., p. 138.

GROUP PRAYER REQUESTS   TODAY'S DATE:_____

NAME	REQUEST	RESULTS

A BIG GOAL AND LIFE CONTROL

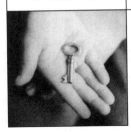

MEMORY VERSE

May God himself, the God of peace,
sanctify you through and through. May your
whole spirit, soul and body be kept blameless
at the coming of the Lord Jesus Christ.
1 Thessalonians 5:23

Several years ago, an investment company ran a television ad that contained this line: "The day cannot begin early enough for the man consumed by a single goal in life."

During these last weeks of this study, you've focused on some specific goals for weight control and health. The goals are significant, but your long-term success depends on how well you fit your First Place goals into broader life goals.

In this week's study, you'll read about the life of the apostle Paul. You'll learn how he continually relied on God to sanctify him. He kept himself blameless for the Lord Jesus Christ. You'll have an opportunity to think about your own goals and how they fit into God's plan.

DAY 1: *Living with a Purpose*

Oliver Wendell Holmes once said, "The greatest thing in this world is not so much where we are, but in what direction we are moving." Some goals describe the destination. Other goals become the map that charts the route between where you are and where you want to be.

➣ In 1 Thessalonians 5:23, Paul asked for the God of peace to sanctify him. He told the Thessalonians to keep their whole spirit, soul and body blameless before the Lord. What did he mean by this?

God wants you as His for a reason. In His design, you fit into His plan. Part of the adventure in life is discovering His plan and sensing the potential that you have in Him. Never should you become negative and discouraged about your life. Whether or not you admit it, the truth is that God saw value and potential in your life. Your task is to see yourself as He sees you—not as you are, but as you will become! He wants to sanctify You and make you in His image.

Paul's purpose in life was to know Jesus Christ. He was excited about the things that Christ was doing in him. But his primary focus was in knowing Christ and serving Him and thus to be blameless before Him. In Philippians 3:7-11, Paul said that compared to knowing Christ, everything else is rubbish! After reading this passage in Philippians, complete the phrases below:

➤ Gain Christ and be _____ in Him.

➤ Obtain the _____ that is by faith.

➤ Know Christ and the _____ of His resurrection.

➤ Know Christ in the _____ of His sufferings.

➤ Become like Christ in His _____.

➤ Attain to the _____ from the dead.

➤ Could you say, with Paul, that knowing Christ and experiencing the things listed in the phrases you just completed are the most important focus of your life? Why?

Heavenly Father, help me be blameless before You by knowing You more fully. For Your sake I consider everything a loss compared to the surpassing greatness of knowing Christ Jesus, my Lord.

When the Roman army conquered an enemy, soldiers sometimes strapped the bodies of the dead onto the backs of the prisoners and forced them to carry the corpse as it decomposed. This practice would disgust us, yet many people today strap painful memories of past failure onto their lives and carry them, allowing the past to obstruct their future. Fortunately, in Christ, past sin can be forgiven. More than that, past failure can provide motivation for positive future living. The word "sanctify" means to be free from sin. When you accepted Christ as your Savior, He freed you from those past sins.

Paul refers to God as a God of peace. He gives a peace that goes beyond our understanding when we trust in Him as Paul did.

➣ According to Romans 8:6, what was the source of Paul's peace?

When Paul became a Christian, he didn't have spiritual amnesia about his past. He always remembered how he had persecuted Christians. Since Christ had forgiven him, he used his past as a testimony of Jesus' love and forgiveness. He allowed God to sanctify him for service in obedience to His commands.

One definition of "sanctify" is to set apart, make holy, consecrate. This was Paul's desire throughout his ministry. God forgave him of the things he had done and set him apart to preach and teach God's Word to the world. He could not have done this without God's peace.

God Himself is the One at work in you and through you. Beth Moore tells us that "He hasn't just assigned you a mighty angel. God is thoroughly interested and involved in every single part of you: body, soul, and spirit."[1]

Do you recall the memory verse for week 2? In that Scripture, God is described as the God of hope who will fill you with all peace. Isn't it natural to believe that if God is peace, He will give you peace?

How has God given you peace when your life has been in turmoil?

Lord, thank You for being faithful and just in forgiving my sin and purifying me from all unrighteousness.

Thank You, Father, for Your work in me and through me and for being interested and involved in every part of me.

DAY 3: *Being Sanctified to Be Free from Sin*

Accepting Christ as your personal Savior sets you free from your past sins. His Spirit takes up residence in yours and sets you apart.

What does 1 Corinthians 6:17 tell you about the Holy Spirit?

Beth Moore says that "the key to victory . . . is to bow daily . . . to the control of the Holy Spirit over your body."[2] God wants to have control over every part of your being—spirit, mind, soul and body. If you let Him control only one or two parts, you will miss the full meaning and joy of His peace.

What does Colossians 3:15 instruct you to do?

The peace of Christ comes when He is in full control of every part of your life. The soul represents the heart of your emotions and feelings and personality. When you let any one part control your life—such as eating habits, negative attitudes or out-of-control feelings—you distance yourself from the God of peace. You let your physical appetite and drives take over, and they become the authority by which you live.

⇨ What good advice does Paul give in Colossians 3:5 about your earthly nature?

⇨ According to Colossians 3:12, how are you to clothe yourself as one of God's chosen?

⇨ How does this impact you personally?

⇨ Once you submit your whole being to God's control, you can claim the promise set forth in Philippians 4:7. Write the promise in your own words.

 God, I live every minute of my life in Your presence, and I am ultimately accountable to You. Help me live to please You.

Thank You, Father, for being a God of hope and peace. Let me worship You with every part of my being.

DAY 4: *Being Faithful to the End*

Since Paul's goal in life was to know Christ and live life to please Him, nothing in life could stop Paul. He set his mind on being kept blameless at the coming of Christ. More than anything else in life, Paul wanted to experience Christ in every part of his being. He understood what Christ had done for him. He remembered his sin for which Christ had died.

In his letters to the church at Thessalonica, Paul urged the Christians to encourage each other as they served God.

➤ In 1 Thessalonians 5:14-18, what did Paul tell them to do?

➤ Of what benefit are these actions?

When Christians encourage and build each other up, they help others to keep themselves blameless and right with God.

Although the words "soul" and "spirit" are many times used interchangeably in Scripture, there is a distinct separation in many verses. The spirit is thought of as being conscious of the existence of God and able to communicate with God, while the soul is the seat of the affections, desires, emotions and will. Thus, these two along with the body make up our whole beings. Paul stated that all three are to be kept blameless.

➤ According to Romans 8:6, what is the reward of one whose mind is controlled by the Spirit?

Do you feel the peace of God through your entire being? If not, then surrender today to His wise, loving and freedom-giving authority. He wants to make you clean, pure and totally devoted to Him. He wants to set you apart for a special use.

Heavenly Father, help me to be totally surrendered to You so that You can use my life for Your special service.

Father God, I bow before You in complete humility and recognize You as the one true God.

DAY 5: *Focusing on a Big Goal for Life*

Spiritual goals can lead to positive life control. As you seek to know
Christ and live for Him, that overarching goal will focus on Christ in such
a way that His work in you can proceed without hindrance. As you know
Christ more fully, you begin to live with His perspective, His power and
His character. Knowing Christ is the key to achieving every other goal in
your life. Someone once said, "The main thing is make sure the main
thing is the main thing." For the Christian, the main life goal should be
knowing Christ—not success, not accomplishment, not weight control.
When Christ becomes the main thing in your life, other things fall into
perspective and you can deal with them in Christ's power. As the God of
peace sanctifies you through and through, your desire will be to stay fully
devoted to Him and in His service.

⇝ What can you do in your daily life to keep yourself ready for service?

⇝ If you continue to live as you do now, will you experience God's
peace?

⇝ How can the commitments in the First Place program help you live
for Him?

Paul wrote to the Thessalonians to urge them to keep themselves
blameless for the coming of the Lord. He knew what was involved in living a blameless life and keeping himself ready for Christ's return. He
suffered many hardships and obstacles, but he persevered and knew his
life was ready for the return of Jesus Christ.

➤ From 2 Corinthians 11:23-29, list the types of hardships and obstacles endured by Paul after becoming a Christian.

➤ Which hardships endured by Paul might have made you give up?

With God's help you can endure any hardship or obstacle Satan may put in your life. Satan wants you to fail. He wants you to give up and forsake your goals. Let God take over and give you victory. He is ready and waiting for you to ask Him.

Thank You, Father, for being faithful to Your Word and giving me Your peace.

Dear Lord, help me to fix my eyes on You and to live a life pleasing to You.

DAY 6: *Reflections*

As you strive to be blameless before God, you know you will face obstacles and have to overcome strongholds in your life. Remember that the definition of a stronghold is anything that sets itself up as better than God or goes against the knowledge of God. No matter whether the stronghold is physical or emotional, you have the weapons of divine power to demolish those strongholds.

Prayer and the Word of God are two of your most powerful weapons to help you stay on course. Satan will flee in the presence of prayer and Scripture. Think about the things that come into your everyday life that may be a stumbling block or could become a stronghold. In *Praying God's Word*, Beth Moore explains how to overcome strongholds.[3]

Each week your lessons have stressed the importance of memorizing Scriptures and quoting them as you pray or encourage others. The Bible contains verses that meet every need a person could ever have. When the verses are hidden in your heart, you have the tools at hand to face every struggle that comes your way, every temptation Satan can give you and every stronghold that threatens to undermine you.

The following are prayers based on Scripture that will give you hope and power:

Lord God, help me to never be lacking in zeal, but help me keep my spiritual fervor as I serve You; and help me be joyful in hope, patient in affliction and faithful in prayer (see Romans 12:11-12).

Father God, I thank You for everything that was written in the past to teach me so that through endurance and the encouragement of the Scriptures, I might have hope (see Romans 15:4).

Thank You, Lord, for giving me weapons, not of this world, but weapons that have divine power to demolish strongholds (see 2 Corinthians 10:4).

DAY 7: *Reflections*

As you come to the end of this First Place session, you may be evaluating your goals and what you have accomplished during this time. How do you measure the success you have had in the program? Do you measure strictly by pounds lost, or do you look at the overall picture and evaluate your spiritual growth? Which is more important: to please others or to please God?

If you have memorized Bible verses, prayed for fellow class members, studied your Bible regularly and participated by coming to the meetings, sharing your needs and sharing your insights in the Bible study, you have been successful in growing spiritually. If you have had problems in any of these areas and did not succeed as you would have liked, you are not a failure. You simply haven't reached your goals in the time you set. Keep working, keep reading the Bible, keep praying and stay the course. God's plans don't always include immediate success. He sometimes asks you to wait, so continue to follow His will and He will lead you to success.

Your leader(s) will continue to pray for you and wish you the very best as you continue in your endeavors to seek God and let Him give you a life under His control. You have been given the weapons to fight your battles against Satan. Use them in your daily walk as you encounter any obstacle that threatens to undermine your efforts to have a closer relationship with God.

 Heavenly Father, help me to forget what is behind and strain toward what is ahead as I press on toward the goal to win the prize for which You have called me heavenward in Christ Jesus (see Philippians 3:13-14).

O God, never let me show contempt for the riches of Your kindness, tolerance and patience. Help me realize that Your kindness leads me toward repentance (see Romans 2:4).

Father, Your Word assures me that it is You who works in me to will and to act according to Your good purpose (see Philippians 2:13).

God of peace, sanctify me through and through. May my spirit, soul and body be kept blameless at the coming of our Lord Jesus Christ (see 1 Thessalonians 5:23).

Notes
1. Beth Moore, *Praying God's Word* (Nashville, TN: Broadman and Holman Publishers, 2000), p. 89.
2. Ibid., p. 150.
3. Ibid., pp. 2-3.

Group Prayer Requests   Today's Date:_____

Name	Request	Results

DINING *DELIZIOSO!*

Italian food is an American favorite! Almost everyone has a favorite little Italian restaurant. Typically serving good food and having quaint atmospheres, Italian restaurants are a great place to fellowship with family and friends. Italian food offers many healthy choices. Fresh breads, pastas and tomato-based sauces are great choices on any eating plan. But depending on how they're prepared, these same foods can be less healthy choices: garlic bread with butter and cheese, pastas cooked in oil or covered with cheese, cream-based sauces and large portions. Add the cheesecake and you can easily exceed a day's worth of calories.

A Taste of Italy

You may not speak Italian, but you can learn how to read the menu. Learn these common terms to help you make more healthful choices:

Low in fat	High in Fat
Baked, broiled or roasted	*Alfredo*—butter or cheese sauces
Primavera	*Crema*—cream-based sauces
Marinara—tomato-based sauces	*Fritto*—fried
Marsala or *cacciatore*	Garlic bread
Red or white clam sauce	*Parmigiana*
Minestrone	Cheese- or meat-filled pastas

Pesto—just because it's green doesn't mean it's low fat!
Pesto, made with basil, olive oil, pine nuts and grated cheese, is generally high in fat and calories. Use it carefully!

Healthy Choices for Any Occasion

Appetizers
How does hot garlic bread sound? Be careful—a couple of slices can add up to 500 calories! Ask that your waiter not bring the garlic bread to the

table, or plan to split a piece with a companion. Dipping your bread in olive oil also adds calories. Ask for bread without the butter, or have bread sticks instead.

Start your meal with minestrone soup or gazpacho and a salad with dressing on the side. You can even make these your main meal. A Caesar salad with eggs, creamy dressing, grated cheese and croutons is generally high in fat and calories.

Do you enjoy antipasto? Antipasto with seafood and marinated vegetables is usually your best choice. Watch out for antipasto with lots of cheese, fried vegetables, meats and olives, all of which can be high in calories and fat.

The Main Meal

Italian portions are often two to three times more than you need. Remember a serving of pasta is a half cup! Ask for a to-go box before your meal and keep the extra portions for another day. You could also split a dish with a companion.

Choose the following dishes for a healthier meal:

- Grilled chicken breast or veal with marsala or cacciatore
- Pasta with marinara or pasta primavera (pasta with vegetables)
- Clam sauce

Avoid the following:

- Lasagna or cheese-filled pasta (ravioli, cannelloni and manicotti)
- Italian sausage, pancetta (bacon) or prosciutto (ham)
- Eggplant or veal parmigiana—breaded and fried

Other Tips to Remember

Let family or friends who are dining with you know that you plan to eat healthy. Order what you know is best for you, and don't let others tempt you into ordering less healthy choices. Make a plan and stick with it. Remember your goal of reaching or maintaining a healthy weight.

Become familiar with a few restaurants you enjoy and where you know you can order healthy foods. Learn to make special requests like substituting tomato-based sauces for cream- or cheese-based sauces. Ask that your meal be prepared with less oil or butter. Avoid restaurants and foods that can knock you off your plan.

What About Pizza?

Pizza can be a healthy choice. Here are some tips for ordering:

- Order a thin-crust pizza instead of thick-crust or deep-dish.
- Ask that the pizza be prepared with less or even no cheese.
- Top the pizza with fresh vegetables instead of high-fat and high-sodium meats.
- Limit yourself to one or two pieces; for added variety eat a salad instead of an extra piece.

In the following table, list the Italian restaurants where you dine most often. Next, list the foods that you usually order. Now what can you do to make your meals healthier? Use this table to help you plan for healthy choices the next time you eat Italian food.

Restaurant	Usual Choices (be specific)	Better Choices

MORE FACTS ABOUT FAT

ALL FATS ARE NOT CREATED EQUAL

In terms of calories, all fats are created equal—nine calories per gram. The difference is the effect specific fats have on cholesterol levels and other aspects of health. You're probably aware that diets high in saturated fat and cholesterol are associated with higher levels of blood cholesterol and greater risk for heart disease. Certain cancers may also be related to higher intakes of saturated fat. Certain fats—in moderation—may even have beneficial effects on health. Monounsaturated fatty acids in olive and canola oils may increase HDL (*good*) cholesterol in some people when substituted for saturated fat in the diet.

Because not all fats are created equal when it comes to health, it's important to pay attention to the types of fat you eat. No one is recommending that you increase the amount of fat in your eating plan, but it is important to shift the balance in favor of healthier fats.

Experts recommend the following limitations:

- Total fat to 30 percent or less of calories
- Saturated fat to less than 10 percent of calories
- Polyunsaturated fat to 10 percent of calories
- Monounsaturated fat to between 10 percent and 15 percent of calories

RATING THE OILS

Fats and oils contain a combination of all three types of fatty acids: saturated, polyunsaturated and monounsaturated. All oils are 100 percent fat and contain 120 calories per tablespoon. The following chart compares fats higher in unsaturated fatty acids with those higher in saturated fatty acids.

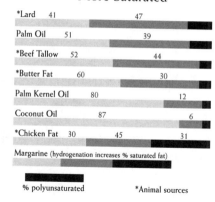

More Unsaturated		More Saturated	
Safflower Oil 13	70	*Lard 41	47
Sunflower Oil 20	69	Palm Oil 51	39
Soybean Oil 24	61	*Beef Tallow 52	44
Cottonseed Oil 19	54	*Butter Fat 60	30
Corn Oil 25	62	Palm Kernel Oil 80	12
Peanut Oil 48	34	Coconut Oil 87	6
Canola Oil 58	36	*Chicken Fat 30 45	31
Olive Oil 77	9	Margarine (hydrogenation increases % saturated fat)	

% saturated   % monounsaturated   % polyunsaturated   *Animal sources

The following are tips for including fats and oils in a healthy eating plan:

- Cut down on all fats and oils.
- Choose unsaturated sources of fat more often than saturated sources.
- Choose a monounsaturated source such as canola or olive oil, and a polyunsaturated source such as safflower or corn oil. Use limited amounts of both in cooking and preparing foods.
- Choose soft tub margarine with liquid vegetable oil or water listed as the first ingredient more often than margarine (with hydrogenated fats as the first ingredient), stick margarine or butter.

WHAT IS A SERVING OF FAT?

To meet the above guidelines for total fat intake and balance, limit yourself to three to five servings of fat each day. Choose the following unsaturated fats instead of ones higher in saturated fat. One exchange equals:

1 teaspoon vegetable oil	2-3 teaspoons seeds or nuts
1 tablespoon lite margarine	1/8 medium avocado
1 tablespoon lite salad dressing	1 teaspoon peanut butter
1 teaspoon regular mayonnaise	1 teaspoon regular margarine
1 tablespoon lite mayonnaise	5 large or 10 small olives

Remember: A fat exchange equals 5 grams of fat. Watch out for hidden fats in your eating plan!

What About Hydrogenated Fats and Trans Fatty Acids?

You may have heard about hydrogenated fats. Hydrogenation is a process that makes unsaturated oils more solid at room temperature (i.e., more like saturated fats). Hydrogenation also increases the amount of trans fatty acids. Trans fatty acid simply refers to where the hydrogen is placed on the fat molecule. Actually, trans fatty acids are found naturally in many foods such as meat, butter and milk. You will commonly see the terms "partially hydrogenated" or "hydrogenated" vegetable oil on the labels of many processed foods such as margarine, salad dressings, crackers, chips and other baked goods. Hydrogenated fats and trans fatty acids can raise blood cholesterol levels but probably not as much as saturated fats. Choose margarine that lists liquid vegetable oil or water as the first ingredient and no more than two grams of saturated fat per tablespoon. There is no reason to switch to butter because of health concerns about hydrogenated fats or trans fatty acids.

Omega-3 Fatty Acids

Omega-3 fatty acids are polyunsaturated fatty acids found mostly in cold-water fish and some vegetable oils. Omega-3 fatty acids may reduce the risk of heart disease through effects on cholesterol, blood-clotting factors and blood pressure. Good sources include salmon, albacore tuna, mackerel, sardines and lake trout. *Eat more fish!* A healthy eating plan can include several servings each week. Canola, soybean and flaxseed oils are also good sources of omega-3 fatty acids.

Fat-Replacers—Fake Fats

Fat-replacers are added to cheeses, desserts, salad dressings and snack foods to give them the taste and feel of the "full-fat" versions—without the calories! Olestra (OLEAN) is one of the newer fat-replacers. Olestra is made from a combination of vegetable fat and carbohydrate. It's calorie free because it passes through the body without being digested. Olestra appears to be safe, but it may interfere with the absorption of the fat-soluble vitamins and cause digestive discomfort in some people. Simplesse is a fat-replacer found mostly in frozen dairy products. It's made from protein. Although foods made with fat-replacers are low in fat, they still have calories and can be low in nutrients.

As always, moderation, balance and variety are the keys to a healthy eating plan.

OVERCOMING DIFFICULT SITUATIONS

A prudent man foresees difficulty and plans accordingly.
—see Proverbs 27:12

How does it feel to be on the road to change? You should feel good about your efforts! But here is the $10,000 question: Is it as easy as you thought it would be?

Difficult situations, temptations and setbacks are an expected and natural part of making lifestyle changes. Many people envision weight loss as a race that begins with a mad dash down the track and finishes at the line in record time. It's important to know that the road to change has many hurdles and hazards along the way—and it's a lifelong journey! It's important to know your course, set your eye on the prize and run with endurance the race set before you (see Philippians 3:12-14; Hebrews 12:1).

Review the following three-step process and use the following worksheet to help you understand how and when you will be tempted. Most important, use it to develop a plan of attack when temptation strikes or you experience a setback.

STEP 1—IDENTIFY DIFFICULT SITUATIONS

The first step is to know your course and what lies ahead. Start by identifying situations—people, places, feelings and foods—that make it difficult for you to stick with your plan. Think carefully about your behavior. Do you eat when you are lonely or angry or when you feel out of control in other areas of your life? Do you tend to overeat at parties or other social situations? Is there a certain restaurant where you almost always overeat? Talk to family and friends to get a better understanding of those situations that are difficult for you. Review your First Place Fact Sheets to see where you are having the most difficulty. Are you using your Fact Sheets regularly?

STEP 2—UNDERSTAND YOUR USUAL RESPONSE TO DIFFICULT SITUATIONS

Perhaps the most crucial part of any plan is understanding how you respond to difficult situations and slipups. Engrain this in your mind: *Temptation and slipups are an important part of the process of change.* Temptation and slipups are not failures; they're opportunities to learn and move closer to your goal. Unfortunately, because of negative thinking or unrealistic expectations, many people allow a slipup to throw them completely off course. By knowing and understanding your usual responses, you can turn what you think is weakness into strength. How do you usually respond when faced with a difficult situation? Do you often give in to temptation or the influence of others? Do you feel guilty when you make mistakes? Do you feel like a failure? Have slipups knocked you off your program in the past?

STEP 3—DEVELOP A PLAN OF ACTION

After identifying difficult situations and how you typically respond, you can begin to plan a solid defense. A prudent person foresees difficulty and plans accordingly. Having a plan provides you with a road map that will help you stay on course. Make a list of strategies you can use to get you through difficult situations. For example, how can you turn negative thoughts—*Now that I've blown it, what's the use of trying?*—into more positive responses—*What went wrong here; how can I avoid this next time?* Don't forget the importance of enlisting support. Friends and family are a great source of help and encouragement—use them!

- Ask your spouse to drop off or pick up the children so you can work out.
- Give your friends a list of restaurants that make it easy for you to stick to your eating plan.
- Find someone to walk with you during your lunch break three times a week.
- Find an accountability partner to check in with once a week.

Copy this worksheet and keep it with you for the next several weeks. Review your First Place Commitment Records to find your areas of difficulty. Write down as many things as you can about situations that are difficult for you and how you usually respond to them. Begin thinking of ways to respond differently—*What will I do?*—the next time you face a similar situation. What things can you do to help you stay on track?

Difficult Situation (person, place, feeling, and food)	How Do I Usually Respond?	What Will I Do?

KEEP YOUR EYE ON THE PRIZE

Remember, your goal is to eat healthfully for a lifetime and to gradually achieve your healthy weight. Take time to understand yourself and what circumstances make it difficult for you to reach and maintain your goals. Most people are in such a hurry to reach their goals that they fail to plan for difficult situations. People who are successful in making lifestyle changes recognize that setbacks are normal and they plan for them!

Also, they don't see setbacks as failures. They see them as learning opportunities they can use to do better next time. It's what we do over weeks and months that makes the difference in our health and quality of life. If you slip up one day, the next day just pick right up where you left off.

It's also important to reward yourself and feel good about the progress you're making along the way. Recognize and celebrate your success. Lifestyle change and healthier habits bring real benefits. Personal rewards such as feeling better, having more energy, better self-esteem and improved health are the strongest motivators. You're more likely to stick with your program if it makes you feel good. You can reward yourself in other ways too. A new outfit, a night out on the town or a weekend getaway are also ways you can reward yourself. Contract with a loved one or friend for special rewards along the way.

➤ What are some ways you can be rewarded for your efforts?

In this whole process of change, remember who is on your side.

If the LORD delights in a man's way, he makes his steps firm; though he stumble, he will not fall, for the LORD upholds him with his hand.
—Psalm 37:23-24

OVERCOMING OBSTACLES TO PHYSICAL ACTIVITY

No, in all these things we are more than conquerors
through him who loved us.
—Romans 8:37

Most of us don't need to be told that physical activity is good for us. While knowing why and how to become more physically active is important, the more important question is, *How can I get started and then stick with it?* Have you been physically active in the past and then stopped? You're not alone; more than 50 percent of people who start an exercise program drop out within the first three to six months. By the end of a year only one out of four are still active. There are many reasons people give for not starting or sticking with a physical activity program. By making yourself aware of your personal obstacles to physical activity, you can improve your chances of sticking with your program for a lifetime.

See if you recognize yourself in the following list of excuses, and then read the helpful solutions:

I DON'T ENJOY EXERCISE

Don't exercise. Find physical activities you enjoy—try a sport or active hobby. Find someone to exercise with you. Listen to music, pray or find other ways to take your mind off the activity.

I DON'T HAVE TIME FOR EXERCISE

You have to make time—30 minutes several days a week is all it takes. Break up your activity into shorter segments of 5, 10 or 15 minutes. Schedule activity just like you would any other important meeting. Ask family and friends to help you make the time.

I'm Too Tired to Exercise

Low energy levels are often the result of low fitness and too much stress; regular physical activity improves fitness, increases energy levels and is a great stress reliever.

Exercise Is Not Convenient

Physical activity can be done anywhere and anytime. Look for opportunities to fit physical activity into your day—walk during your lunch break, buy home exercise equipment, find a health club nearby. Community centers, YMCAs, colleges and some churches have fitness facilities that are convenient and affordable.

Exercise Is Too Hard

Activity doesn't have to be hard to be beneficial. The important thing is that you choose activities you enjoy. Many people want quick results, so they start off doing too much too soon.

I Don't Have Anyone to Exercise with Me

Maybe you're not asking enough people; ask family, friends, neighbors, coworkers and church acquaintances. Join a sports or recreation group. Check with community centers, colleges and local fitness clubs.

I Don't Feel Any Different When I Exercise

Don't expect to feel good right away. It takes time for your body to adapt to regular physical activity. After four to six weeks of regular activity, you should start feeling and seeing a difference. Monitor your progress along the way.

I'm Too Overweight and Out of Shape

Physical activity and good health have nothing to do with the way you look or how well you perform; it's about being the best you can be. Never compare yourself to others. Always remember that you're truly fearfully and wonderfully made (see Psalm 139:14)! Choose activities you enjoy and do them in a comfortable environment. Don't let your feelings about yourself or your perceptions about what other people think keep you from achieving your goals.

I Don't Have Any Reason to Be Active

Find reasons! Prayerfully consider the benefits of living a more physically active lifestyle—reduced risk of heart disease, cancer, diabetes, high blood pressure and osteoporosis, more energy, weight loss and maintenance, improved mood, higher quality of life. The stronger your motivations, the more likely you'll be successful. Read Mark 12:28-31; Psalm 139:14 and 1 Corinthians 6:19-20. How do these verses speak of the importance of taking good care of yourself? When we are physically fit, we can better serve the Lord.

The Weather Is Bad

Get out of the habit of using weather as an excuse for not being physically active. With the appropriate clothing and gear, you can enjoy activity all year long. If you can't get outside, work out in your home, walk in the mall or join a fitness center.

My Family and Friends Are Not Supportive

Family and friends who aren't supportive can make it very difficult. The key is communication. Find creative ways to get others involved in your program. Surround yourself with others who are more supportive. Be sensitive to others, but don't allow them to sabotage your efforts. Get out there and do it anyway, and maybe when they see the benefits, they'll be motivated to join you!

Exercise Seems So Self-Centered

In the Bible study, you've read that you are God's good creation and your body is the temple of the Holy Spirit. You're responsible for caring for your body. A physically active lifestyle and the benefits it brings will give you the energy you need for effective living and serving others. The focus of your activity should be on caring for your body and honoring God.

What are *your* obstacles? You need to anticipate that you will have difficulties. Things will interfere with your ability and desire to exercise. The key is to expect the obstacles, plan ahead and make a commitment to stick with your goals.

What is keeping you from being active now? What obstacles are most likely to interfere with your physical activity program? How can you get back on track if you stop? Make sure your obstacles are not just excuses. We find the time and the ways to do the things that are important to us. Learn to turn negative thinking into positive: *I can, I will, I'm willing to try*.

OVERCOMING STRESS

Do not be anxious about anything, but in everything,
by prayer and petition, with thanksgiving, present your requests to God.
And the peace of God, which transcends all understanding,
will guard your hearts and minds in Christ Jesus.

—Philippians 4:6-7

Do you ever feel like the treadmill of life is stuck on high speed and there's no one around to slow it down? Are the pressures of work, home, finances and other responsibilities piling up so fast, you often wonder if you can keep up? Do you feel like you're being pushed and pulled in so many different directions that you think you might break in two? Do you feel like there's just no time for *you*? Are you having a hard time experiencing the abundant life that Christ desires for you (see John 10:10)? If you can identify (and you probably can) with any of these questions, you're probably stressed.

WHAT IS STRESS?

First, it's important to understand that stress is not an event or circumstance—it's our response to an event or circumstance. Stress is the response of our bodies or minds to physical or emotional strain, such as overwork or too much worry. From a biblical standpoint, stress or worry means to divide the mind and it occurs when you take your focus off that which is truly important. Some experts refer to stress as "hurry sickness."

Fortunately, God has given us the ability to recognize and respond to challenges. The stress response protects us and allows us to persevere against the Goliaths of life. The body responds to challenges by releasing a number of hormones, such as adrenaline, which rev up the body and prepare it for action. Stress experts refer to this response as "fight or flight." David had a choice whether to fight or run from Goliath. Unfortunately, many of our battles pile up faster than we can keep up, and it's much harder to run from deadlines, traffic jams and bills. In fact, much of our stress is caused by thinking about things that haven't yet happened— and probably never will, such as worrying that a loved one will be involved in an accident. Over time, the stress response begins to take its toll on the body, mind and spirit.

THE HARMFUL EFFECTS OF STRESS

Our bodies—God's temple—are clearly not designed for chronic stress. Stress is linked to heart disease, high blood pressure, obesity, depression and unhealthy habits. Stress causes headaches, backaches and digestive problems. Chronic stress suppresses the immune system and makes the body susceptible to a variety of illnesses. Stress can make you feel angry, irritable, afraid, excited or helpless. Stress makes it hard to sleep or relax, and it leaves you feeling fatigued. It's no wonder that God's Word repeatedly tells us not to worry or be anxious (see Matthew 6:25; John 14:27; Philippians 4:6-7). In fact, it has been said that you can't worry and trust in God at the same time.

➤ Is stress or excessive worry affecting your health and quality of life? How?

➤ How is stress affecting your relationship with God or important people in your life?

To find out if you are stressed, circle yes or no in answer to each of the following questions:

Do you often feel tense, nervous or anxious?   Yes No
Do you have a hard time relaxing or turning off your thoughts? Yes No

Do you often worry about all the things you have to do?	Yes	No
Do you have a hard time concentrating or staying focused?	Yes	No
Do you often feel like things are out of your control?	Yes	No
Do you constantly feel like you're in a hurry?	Yes	No
Do you notice that you're irritable or getting angry often?	Yes	No
Do you often take on more than you can handle?	Yes	No

If you answered yes to one or more of these questions, chances are that stress is taking its toll on your health and quality of life. Are you ready to learn some ways to change your response to the challenges of your life?

A BIBLICAL PLAN FOR TAMING THE STRESS RESPONSE

TRUST IN GOD

> Trust in the LORD with all your heart and lean not on your own understanding; in all your ways acknowledge him, and he will make your paths straight (Proverbs 3:5-6).

Do you view life from God's perspective? Have you gotten out of touch with God and His purpose for your life? Whose strength do you rely on when you're faced with a challenge or you're feeling overwhelmed? Stress is a signal to return your focus to God. When you're feeling stressed, re-member that God loves you and is in control of all things.

OVERCOME STRESS THROUGH PRAYER

> Do not be anxious about anything, but in everything, by prayer and petition, with thanksgiving, present your requests to God (Philippians 4:6).

➤ What happens to your prayer life during times of stress?

➻ According to Philippians 4:7, what will be the result of your prayers during times of stress and worry?

Never underestimate the power of prayer in dealing with the challenges of life. Learn to listen to the Lord and He will provide a way out for you.

Focus on What Is Most Important

> Finally, brothers, whatever is true, whatever is noble, whatever is right, whatever is pure, whatever is lovely, whatever is admirable—if anything is excellent or praiseworthy—think about such things (Philippians 4:8).

In times of stress, ask yourself if your mind is set on the truth. Are you realistically evaluating and responding to your situation? Are you applying your mind to positive solutions?

Take Positive Steps to Change the Situation

> Whatever you have learned or received or heard from me, or seen in me—put it into practice. And the God of peace will be with you (Philippians 4:9).

The key to dealing with stress is to take positive action. Nothing is ever changed by worry. Identify the source of your stress and begin taking steps to either eliminate it or deal with it in positive ways.

PREVENTING CANCER

Scientific evidence suggests that nearly 30 percent of cancer deaths are related to dietary factors. In fact, experts predict that for the majority of Americans who don't smoke, dietary and physical activity habits are the most important modifiable risk factors for cancer. There is little doubt that nutrition plays a role in contributing to and preventing cancer. A definitive answer about the optimal diet for preventing cancer and which nutrients have specific effects is not yet known.

What Is Cancer?

Cancer is a group of diseases caused by the abnormal growth and spread of the body's cells. When these cells grow out of control, they can develop into cancerous (malignant) tumors. Cancers result in death by interfering with several of the body's normal processes.

Many factors contribute to cancer, including heredity, aging, environment and lifestyle. For example, a smoker's risk of developing lung cancer is 10 times higher than that of a nonsmoker. A woman with a mother, sister or daughter with breast cancer has about twice the risk of developing breast cancer compared to a woman who does not have such a family history. Too much exposure to the sun's rays increases the risk for skin cancer. Early detection and eliminating risk factors are very important aspects of preventing cancer and cancer deaths.

Cancer and Nutritional Health

Several groups publish nutrition guidelines to advise the public about dietary practices that reduce risk of cancer. Current recommendations are based on the consensus of hundreds of experts and thousands of scientific studies. The following are consistent with dietary recommendations from the American Cancer Society, National Cancer Institute, World Cancer Research Fund and the American Institute for Cancer Research:

◉ **Choose most of the foods you eat from plant sources.**

Eat five or more servings of fruits and vegetables each day. Especially try to choose dark green and yellow vegetables, vegetables in the cabbage family, soy products and legumes.

Eat 6 to 11 servings a day of grains including breads, cereals, rice and pasta. Choose mostly whole grains instead of highly processed or refined grains.

◉ **Limit your intake of high-fat foods, particularly those from animal sources.**

Select lean cuts and smaller portions when you eat meat, use low-fat cooking techniques, select nonfat or low-fat dairy products and replace high-fat foods with fruits, vegetables, grains and legumes.

◉ **Get 30 minutes or more of moderate-intensity activity on most days each week.**

◉ **Achieve and maintain a healthy weight.**

◉ **Limit consumption of alcoholic beverages—if you drink at all.**

SCIENTIFIC EVIDENCE

◉ Fruits and vegetables contain over 100 beneficial vitamins, minerals, fiber and phytochemicals (plant chemicals), many of which may protect against cancer. Some of the nutrients that may be specifically beneficial include the antioxidant vitamins, fiber, calcium, folate, selenium, carotenoids, flavinoids and sulfurophanes. Studies show that an increased consumption of fruits and vegetables reduces the risk of certain types of cancer. The evidence is particularly strong for colon cancer.

◉ High-fat diets, particularly saturated fats, are associated with an increase in the risk of cancers of the colon and rectum, prostate and endometrium (uterus).

- Consumption of meat, particularly red meat, has been associated with certain cancers. What's the best advice? Limit meat intake to the recommended servings and portion sizes (three to six ounces); choose lean cuts of meat, poultry (without the skin), fish and meat alternatives such as legumes instead of high-fat red meats; and avoid charring meat over a direct flame.
- Physical activity may help protect against cancer of the colon, breast, prostate and endometrium. The protective effects may be related to energy balance and effects on hormone levels.
- Obesity also appears to increase the risk of developing certain cancers.
- Alcoholic beverages are associated with an increased risk of cancer in the oral cavity, esophagus, larynx and breast.

CANCER SCREENING

Cancer screening is one of the most important steps you can take to increase your chances of surviving cancer. Regular screening examinations are currently recommended for the breast, cervix, colon, oral cavity, prostate, rectum, testes and skin. Self-examinations of the breast, testes and skin are important steps in detecting cancer early. A regular medical checkup can also detect cancers of the thyroid, lymph nodes, ovaries and other areas of the body. Here is a cancer-related checkup schedule recommended by the American Cancer Society:

- **Breast**: Monthly self-examination beginning at age 20. Clinical examination every three years in women aged 20 to 40 and yearly after age 40. The American Cancer Society recommends yearly mammograms beginning at age 40. Some groups recommend at least one mammogram between the ages of 40 and 50 and yearly beginning at age 50. Talk to your doctor about what is best for you.
- **Cervical**: Yearly Pap test and pelvic examination beginning at age 18 (or with the initiation of sexual activity).
- **Colon and Rectum**: Regular screening should begin at age 50 (earlier in people at higher risk). Tests usually involve a yearly examination for blood in the stool and a rectal examination. Every 5 to 10 years a test to look at the inside of the colon should also be performed: sigmoidoscopy, colonoscopy or barium enema. Talk to your doctor about the screening test

and schedule that is best for you. If you have a strong family history of colon cancer or polyps, you may need to begin screening earlier.

◉ **Prostate**: Yearly digital rectal examination and Prostate-Specific Antigen (PSA) beginning at age 50. African-Americans and men with a strong family history of cancer may want to begin screening earlier. Talk to your doctor about what's best for you.

FIRST PLACE
MENU PLANS

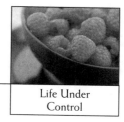

Each plan is based on approximately 1400 calories.

Breakfast	2 breads, 1 fruit, 1 milk, 0-½ fat (When a meat exchange is used, milk is omitted.)
Lunch	2 meats, 2 breads, 1 vegetable, 1 fruit, 1 fat
Dinner	3 meats, 2 breads, 2 vegetables, 1 fat
Snacks	1 bread, 1 fruit, 1 milk, ½-1 fat (or any remaining exchanges)

For more calories, add the following to the 1400 calorie plan.

1600 calories	2 breads, 1 fat
1800 calories	2 meats, 3 breads, 1 vegetable, 1 fat
2000 calories	2 meats, 4 breads, 1 vegetable, 3 fats
2200 calories	2 meats, 5 breads, 1 vegetable, 1 fruit, 5 fats
2400 calories	2 meats, 6 breads, 2 vegetables, 1 fruit, 6 fats

The exchanges for these meals were calculated using the MasterCook software. It uses a database of over 6,000 food items prepared using United States Department of Agriculture (USDA) publications and information from food manufacturers. As with any nutritional program, MasterCook calculates the nutritional values of the recipes based on ingredients. Nutrition may vary due to how the food is prepared, where the food comes from, i.e., geography, soil content, season, ripeness, processing and method of preparation. For these reasons, please use the recipes and menu plans as approximate guides. As always consult your physician and/or a registered dietician before starting a diet program.

🍎 BREAKFASTS

Turkey bacon and egg sandwich:
  2 slices diet whole-wheat bread, toasted; topped with 1 egg, cooked in
      a nonstick pan; and 1 strip turkey bacon, cooked crisp
  1 medium apple
Exchanges: 1 meat, 1 bread, 1 fruit, 1 fat

~~~~~~

  2 low-fat Eggo waffles
  ½ c. unsweetened applesauce to top waffle
  1 pkg. Sweet 'N Low to sprinkle on waffles
  2 tbsp. raisins to top applesauce
  1 cup skim milk
Exchanges: 2 breads, 2 fruits, 1 milk, 1/2 fat

~~~~~~

  1 pkg. flavored instant oatmeal
  3 walnut halves, chopped
  ½ medium-sized banana
  1 c. skim milk
Exchanges: 2 breads, 1 fruit, 1 milk, ½ fat

~~~~~~

  1 medium reduced-fat blueberry muffin
  1 medium fresh peach
  1 c. fruit-flavored yogurt, nonfat and artificially sweetened
Exchanges: 2 breads, 1 fruit, 1 milk, ½ fat

~~~~~~

  ¾ cup Rice Chex cereal
  ½ English muffin
  1 tsp. all-fruit spread
  1 c. skim milk
  ½ banana
Exchanges: 2 breads, 1 fruit, 1 milk

~~~~~~

¼ small cantaloupe or honeydew; topped with 1 cup pineapple-flavored yogurt, nonfat and artificially sweetened

¼ c. Grape Nuts cereal, sprinkled on yogurt

Exchanges: 1 ½ breads, 1 fruit, 1 milk

~~~~~~

1 slice whole-wheat toast or 2 slices diet multigrain toast

2 tsp. all-fruit spread

1 c. nonfat plain or vanilla yogurt with sugar substitute

3 tbsp. wheat germ or 2 tbsp. Grape Nuts cereal

6 oz. calcium-fortified orange juice

Exchanges: 2 breads, 1 fruit, 1 milk

~~~~~~

Brunch Casserole

4 slices wheat bread, crusts removed

2 oz. reduced-fat turkey sausage

¼ c. mushrooms, chopped

1 tsp. onion, chopped

3 eggs, beaten

1 c. skim milk

¼ tsp. salt

⅛ tsp. black pepper

⅛ tsp. granulated garlic

2 oz. reduced-fat cheddar cheese, shredded

Line the bottom of a 9x9-inch casserole dish with the bread. Sauté sausage in a nonstick skillet until done. Remove sausage and sauté mushrooms and onions until tender. Crumble the sausage and combine with the mushrooms and onion. Sprinkle on top of bread. Combine the eggs, milk and seasonings and pour over the bread. Sprinkle with the cheese. Cover and refrigerate overnight. In the morning set out for 15 minutes and then bake at 350° F for 40 to 45 minutes. Cut into four equal portions. Serves 4.

Serve with ½ grapefruit.

Exchanges: 1 ½ meats, 1 bread, 1 fruit, ½ fat

~~~~~~

1 cup Kellogg's Nutri-Grain cereal

1 cup skim milk

2 tbsp. raisins

Exchanges: 2 breads, 1 fruit, 1 milk, ½ fat

~~~~~~

1   6- or 7-inch whole-wheat pocket pita, heated
¼ c. 2% cottage cheese
½ c. canned peaches in their own juice, diced
2   tsp. walnuts, chopped

Combine cottage cheese, peaches and walnuts. Split pita in half and fill each half with ½ of the cottage cheese mixture.
Exchanges: 1 meat, 2 breads, 1 fruit, ½ fat

~~~~~~

Breakfast Burrito

     Vegetable cooking spray
½ c. egg substitute scrambled with:
2   tbsp. onion, chopped
2   tbsp. bell pepper, chopped
2   tbsp. salsa
2   6-inch reduced-fat flour tortillas
     Serve with 1 small orange.
Exchanges: 1 meat, 2 breads, ½ vegetable, 1 fruit, ½ fat

~~~~~~

1   whole 2-oz. wheat bagel
1   tbsp. reduced-fat cream cheese
3   medium stewed prunes or 3 plums
1   c. fat-free milk
Exchanges: 2 breads, 1 fruit, 1 milk, ½ fat

~~~~~~

1   c. oatmeal with dash of cinnamon and nutmeg
2   tbsp. raisins
1   c. fat-free milk
Exchanges: 2 breads, 1 fruit, 1 milk

~~~~~~

3   4-inch low-fat pancakes
6   oz. nonfat plain yogurt
½ c. fresh strawberries, chopped
1   tsp. strawberry all-fruit spread, melted
Combine spread with yogurt and strawberries as pancake topping.
Exchanges: 2 breads, ½ fruit, 1 milk, ½ fat

~~~~~~

Tuna Pocket Sandwich

1 7-inch wheat pita, halved
½ c. romaine lettuce, shredded
½ c. tuna salad
1 tbsp. reduced-calorie mayonnaise
1 tsp. sweet pickle relish

In a small bowl, combine tuna, mayonnaise and pickle relish. Cut the pita in half and stuff lettuce and tuna salad inside each half.

Serve with ½ cup carrot sticks, 1 teaspoon reduced-calorie ranch dressing and 1¼ cups watermelon.
Exchanges: 2 meats, 2 breads, 1 vegetable, 1 fruit, 1 fat

~ ~

Arby's Chicken Sandwich

(regular sliced, no mayonnaise)
    Tossed salad
½ c. celery sticks
2-3 tbsp. reduced-fat salad dressing
1 apple
Exchanges: 2 meats, 2½ breads, 1 vegetable, 1 fruit, 1 fat

~ ~

Ham Muffin

1 English muffin
1 oz. sliced lean ham
    Lettuce and tomato
1 tsp. reduced-fat mayonnaise
½ tsp. mustard
Serve with 1 cup broccoli florets with lite dressing and pear halves (canned in their own juice, drained) filled with ¼ cup 2% cottage cheese.
Exchanges: 2 meats, 2 breads, 1 vegetable, 1 fruit, 1 fat

~ ~

Stouffer's Frozen Lean Cuisine Chicken and Vegetables Vermicelli

Green salad with reduced-fat dressing

1   c. fresh citrus sections

Exchanges: 2 meats, 1 ½ breads, 1 vegetable, 1 fruit, ½ fat

~~~~~~

2   oz. sliced 2% sharp cheddar cheese

8   wheat saltine crackers

1   c. sliced cucumbers, marinated in 1 tbsp. reduced-fat balsamic vinaigrette salad dressing

1   orange

Exchanges: 2 meats, 1 bread, 1 vegetable, 1 fruit, 1 fat

~~~~~~

Peanut Butter Banana Sandwich

2   slices whole wheat bread

1 ½   tbsp. reduced-fat peanut butter

½   banana, sliced

Serve with 1 cup celery sticks with 1 teaspoon reduced-calorie ranch dressing and 1 medium pear.

Exchanges: 2 meats, 2 breads, 1 vegetable, 1 fruit, 1 ½ fats

~~~~~~

Subway Club Sandwich

1   6-inch sandwich made with no added fat or cheese but lots of veggies

1   c. carrot sticks

2   tbsp. lite ranch dressing

15   red grapes

Exchanges: 2 meats, 3 breads, 1 vegetable, 1 fruit, 1 fat

~~~~~~

Stuffed Potato

1   6-oz. baking potato

½   c. cooked broccoli florets

¼   c. sliced mushrooms

1   tbsp. chopped green onions

2   tbsp. 2% cheddar cheese, shredded

1   tbsp. reduced-fat sour cream

Microwave potato until done; then top with cheddar cheese, sour cream, cooked broccoli florets, mushrooms and green onions.

Serve with 1 small banana.

Exchanges: $\frac{1}{2}$ meat, 2 breads, 1 vegetable, 1 fruit, $\frac{1}{2}$ fat

~~~~~~

Pasta Salad

6 oz. uncooked rotini pasta
1 c. celery, sliced
1 c. red bell pepper, sliced
$\frac{1}{4}$ c. onion, chopped
4 oz. feta cheese or Blue cheese, crumbled
4 oz. chicken or turkey, cooked and diced
1 c. cherry tomatoes, halved, for garnish

Dressing:
$\frac{1}{3}$ c. reduced-fat mayonnaise
1 tbsp. Dijon mustard
$\frac{1}{4}$ c. balsamic vinegar
$\frac{1}{4}$ tsp. black pepper
$\frac{1}{8}$ tsp. leaf basil

Cook pasta according to directions. Drain and cool. Mix all dressing ingredients until smooth. Mix pasta with remaining ingredients. Chill before serving. Serves 4.

Exchanges: 2 meats, 2 breads, 1 $\frac{1}{2}$ vegetables, 1 $\frac{1}{2}$ fats per serving

~~~~~~

McDonald's Chef's Salad

1 pkg. Croutons
1 pkg. low-fat dressing
1 small low-fat frozen yogurt cup
1 c. carrot sticks
1 small pear or apple

Exchanges: 2 meats, 2 breads, 2 vegetables, 1 fruit, 1 fat

~~~~~~

Fruited Chicken Salad

8 oz. chicken breast, cooked and diced
$\frac{1}{4}$ c. celery, diced
Mixed lettuce leaves
4 tomatoes, quartered
1 small apple, diced

$\frac{1}{2}$ c. red seedless grapes, halved
$\frac{1}{2}$ c. mandarin orange slices
2 walnut halves, chopped
$\frac{1}{3}$ c. reduced-fat mayonnaise

Combine all ingredients except lettuce and tomatoes. Chill and serve on lettuce with tomatoes. Serves 4.

Serve with 8 wheat crackers per serving.

Exchanges: **2 meats, 1 breads, 1 vegetable, 1 fruit, 1 ½ fats**

~~~~~~

Veggie Pita Sandwich

1	7-inch whole-wheat pita pocket	1	oz. 2% cheddar cheese, sliced
8	cucumber slices	½	tbsp. reduced-fat ranch dressing
4	tomato slices		

Cut pita in half. Divide ingredients in half and fill each half of the pita.

Serve with 1 small apple.

Exchanges: **1 meat, 2 ½ breads, 1 vegetable, 1 fruit, 1 fat**

~~~~~~

Stouffer's Frozen Hearty Portion Lean Cuisine Glazed Chicken with Vegetables and Rice

Serve with 1 small banana.

Exchanges: **2 meats, 2 ½ breads, 1 vegetable, 1 fruit, 1 fat**

~~~~~~

Taco Bell Beef Burrito

Green salad with salsa and reduced-fat sour cream

1   c. carrot sticks

½   c. fresh pineapple, cubed

Exchanges: **2 meats, 3 breads, 1 vegetable, 1 fruit, 1 fat**

~~~~~~

🍎 DINNER

Oven-Fried Chicken

All-Purpose Breading Mix:

1	c. packaged cornflake crumbs	¼	tsp. granulated garlic
1	tsp. paprika	¼	tsp. onion powder
1	tsp. instant chicken bouillon	⅛	tsp. black pepper
½	tsp. poultry seasoning		

Combine all ingredients and mix well. Place in an airtight container. Mix well before using. Makes about 1 cup. Plan on using 2 tablespoons for each chicken breast (you can substitute fish fillet for chicken).
Exchanges: 2 tbsp. = ½ bread

4   4-oz. boneless, skinless chicken breasts
½   c. all-purpose breading
    Vegetable cooking spray

Preheat oven to 425° F. Place breading in a shallow pan. Spray each breast with the cooking spray and coat each side with breading mixture. Arrange in a 9x9-inch baking dish that has been coated with cooking spray. Bake for 15-20 minutes. Serves 4.

Serve each with 1 cup steamed sugar snap peas, a 3-ounce baked potato with 1 teaspoon reduced-fat margarine and 1 teaspoon reduced-fat sour cream.
Exchanges: 3 meats, 1½ breads, 1 vegetable, 1 fat

~~~~~~

Beef Stir-Fry

1 lb. lean beef sirloin	1 c. fresh broccoli florets
1 tsp. chopped garlic	1 c. sliced mushrooms
2 tsp. canola oil	1 tsp. soy sauce
1 red small onion, sliced	3 tbsp. water
1 c. carrots, sliced	4 oz. linguini noodles, uncooked
1 c. zucchini, diced	

Spray a skillet with cooking spray. Add canola oil and heat over high heat. Add beef and stir-fry with garlic until cooked to your liking. Remove and keep warm. Cook noodles without added fat according to package directions. Drain and keep warm. Stir-fry onions and carrots until carrots are partially done. Add water, as needed, to prevent sticking. Add zucchini, broccoli, mushrooms and soy sauce. Stir-fry until vegetables are done to your liking. Add beef to reheat. Toss with pasta and divide into four servings.

Serve with a small breadstick and 1 cup sliced strawberries topped with 1 tablespoon nondairy whipped topping. Any combination of vegetables may be used.
Exchanges: 3 meats, 2 breads, 1 vegetable, 1 fruit, 1 fat

Scallops Parmesan

1 ¼ lb. bay scallops
2 tbsp. reduced-fat margarine
1 28-oz. can diced Italian-style tomatoes, not drained

1 clove garlic, chopped
2 tbsp. lemon juice
¼ c. parmesan cheese, shredded

Over medium-high heat, melt margarine in a skillet. Sauté garlic and scallops for 3 to 4 minutes; add lemon juice and stir. Set aside and keep warm. In a separate skillet cook tomatoes for 5 to 10 minutes, until slightly reduced. Add scallops to tomatoes and heat throughout. Top with parmesan cheese. Serves 4.

Serve each with ½ cup brown rice, 1 cup steamed broccoli and 1 small dinner roll.

Exchanges: 3 meats, 2 breads, 1 ½ vegetables, 1 fat

Salsa Chicken

4 3-oz. boneless, skinless chicken breasts
2 tbsp. Dijon mustard

2 tsp. brown sugar
2 cups chunky salsa
Vegetable cooking spray

Preheat oven to 350° F. Cut each breast into four strips. Arrange chicken in a 9x9-inch baking dish that has been coated with cooking spray. Place chicken in dish and bake uncovered for 10 minutes. Meanwhile combine remaining ingredients in a small dish until well blended. Flip each strip and pour sauce over chicken and bake an additional 8 to 10 minutes or until chicken is done. Serves 4.

Serve each with 1/4 cup reduced-fat refried beans topped with 1 teaspoon part-skim mozzarella cheese and baked, shredded lettuce, diced tomatoes, reduced-fat sour cream and reduced-fat 7-inch flour tortillas.

Exchanges: 3 meats, 2 ½ breads, 1 vegetable, 1 fat

Lemon Fish

1	lb. fish fillets (snapper, tilapia or catfish)	2	tsp. reduced-fat margarine
$\frac{1}{8}$	tsp. black pepper	$\frac{1}{4}$	c. chicken broth
4	lemon slices	$\frac{1}{8}$	tsp. paprika
2	tsp. lemon juice	$\frac{1}{8}$	tsp. dried dill

Arrange fish in a 9x13-inch baking dish. Top with remaining ingredients in order. Bake in a preheated 450° F oven. Bake uncovered for 10 minutes per inch of thickness or until fish flakes easily. Serves 4.

Serve each with $\frac{3}{4}$ cup boiled red potatoes, spinach salad with reduced-fat dressing, $\frac{1}{2}$ cup steamed asparagus with 1 teaspoon melted margarine and 1 dinner roll.

Exchanges: 3 meats, 2 breads, 1 vegetable, 1 fat

~~~~~~

Healthy Choice Frozen Chicken and Pasta Divan

Serve with a tossed salad with 1 tablespoon of reduced-fat dressing and $\frac{1}{2}$ cup fruit salad.

Exchanges: 2 meats, 2$\frac{1}{2}$ breads, 1 vegetable, 1 fruit

~~~~~~

Chicken Curry

1	lb. boneless, skinless chicken breasts, cut into strips	$\frac{1}{2}$	c. raisins
1	tbsp. canola oil	1$\frac{1}{2}$	c. chicken broth, divided
1	tbsp. chopped garlic	2	tbsp. all-purpose flour
1	medium onion, chopped	$\frac{1}{8}$	tsp. black pepper
2	c. Granny Smith apples, diced	$\frac{1}{4}$	tsp. salt (optional)
		1	tbsp. curry

In medium skillet heat oil over medium heat and stir-fry chicken with onion and garlic until chicken is browned. Add curry, apple, raisins, salt (optional) and 1 cup of the broth. Cover and simmer for 10 minutes or until chicken is done. In a covered container, shake flour with remaining broth, or whisk together until there are no lumps. Stir into chicken mixture and bring to a boil, stirring constantly until thickened. Serves 4.

Serve each over $\frac{1}{2}$ cup cooked brown rice, 1 cup cooked green beans and wheat toast points made from sliced diet bread.

Exchanges: 3 meats, 2 breads, 1 vegetable, 1 fruit, 1 fat

Chicken Fajitas

1	lb. boneless, skinless chicken breasts, cut into 1-inch strips	1	green bell pepper, sliced
2	tsp. canola oil	1	medium onion, sliced
3	tbsp. lime juice	8	6-inch reduced-fat flour tortillas
½	tsp. ground cumin	½	c. reduced-fat sour cream
2	c. chunky salsa	½	tsp. chili powder

Mix canola oil, lime juice, cumin and chili powder and pour over chicken. Set aside. Add vegetables to chicken and mix well. Spray a nonstick skillet with cooking spray and stir-fry mixture until done. In a separate skillet, heat tortillas and fill each with chicken mixture. Serve with salsa and sour cream. Makes 4 servings of 2 filled tortillas each.

Exchanges: 3 meats, 2 breads, 1 vegetable, 1 fat

Stuffed Chicken Breasts

4	4-oz. boneless chicken breasts	4	c. packaged seasoned stuffing mix
½	c. onion, chopped	⅛	tsp. black pepper
½	c. celery, chopped	1	can reduced-fat mushroom soup
1½	c. chicken broth	½	c. water
	Vegetable cooking spray		

Preheat oven to 350° F. In a large saucepan, combine onion, celery and broth. Simmer until vegetables are soft. Add stuffing mix and pepper. Mix well and set aside. Place each breast between plastic wrap and pound breast to about ¼ inch thick. Divide stuffing mixture between each breast. Wrap breast around stuffing. Place stuffed breasts in a 9x9-inch pan that has been sprayed with cooking spray. Add ½ cup water to soup and pour over chicken. Bake covered for about 30 minutes or until chicken is no longer pink. Serves 4.

Serve each with 1 cup broccoli slaw.
Exchanges: 3 meats, 2 breads, 2 vegetables, 1 fat

Yogurt Cumin Chicken

4   4-oz. boneless, skinless
    chicken breasts
1   c. green seedless grapes
3   tbsp. all-fruit apricot jam

1   tsp. ground cumin
8   oz. plain nonfat yogurt
    Vegetable cooking spray

Preheat oven to 350° F. Arrange chicken in a 9x9-inch pan that has been coated with cooking spray. Bake uncovered for 20 minutes. Mix yogurt, jam and cumin and spoon over chicken. Bake for an additional 10 minutes. Garnish with grapes prior to serving. Serves 4.

Serve each with baked zucchini and ¾ cup of cooked pasta with ½ cup marinara sauce and 1 dinner roll.

Exchanges: 3 meats, 2½ breads, 2 vegetables, 1 fruit, ½ milk, ½ fat

~~~~~~

Roasted Chicken

Pick up from your favorite store and remove skin before eating. Serves 4.

Serve with ½ cup mashed potatoes and 1 cup Italian green beans and 1 dinner roll with 1 teaspoon of reduced-fat margarine.

Exchanges: 3 meats, 2 breads, 1 vegetable, 1 fat

~~~~~~

Seafood Gumbo

1   lb. mixed seafood (scallops, crab,
    firm fish, deveined shrimp)
1   tsp. garlic, chopped
½   c. onion, chopped
½   c. celery, chopped
½   c. bell pepper, chopped
1   8-oz. pkg. frozen okra
1   28-oz. can stewed tomatoes,
    not drained

Dash cayenne pepper
Tabasco sauce to taste
1   tsp. paprika
2   c. chicken broth, heated
1   tbsp. Worcestershire sauce
1   tbsp. canola oil
4   tbsp. all-purpose flour
½   c. water

In a medium-sized saucepan, sauté onion, celery and bell pepper over medium heat until tender; add garlic and paprika and sauté 1 minute more. Add 1 teaspoon of flour and sauté 2 minutes; do not let burn. Add the heated broth along with the Worcestershire sauce. Bring to a boil, reduce heat and add tomatoes and okra. Let simmer over medium heat until vegetables are tender. Add seasonings. Combine flour with water in a covered container and shake well. Add to gumbo mixture and cook until bubbly. Mixture will thicken. Add seafood and continue to cook until seafood is done. Serves 4.

Serve over ½ cup cooked rice with 1 slice toasted French bread each.
Exchanges: 3 meats, 2 breads, 2 vegetables, 1 fat

~~~~~~

Hearty Beef Stew

¾	lb. lean boneless top-round steak	¼	tsp. dried leaf thyme
2½	tbsp. all-purpose flour		Vegetable cooking spray
⅛	tsp. salt	¾	c. onion, coarsely chopped
⅛	tsp. black pepper	2	tsp. beef-flavored
¾	lb. new potatoes, quartered		bouillon granules
3	stalks celery, cut diagonally	1	28-oz. can stewed tomatoes
	into 1-inch pieces	2	c. water
2	bay leaves	½	tsp. dried sage
2	large carrots, scraped and cut diagonally into 1-inch pieces.		

Trim any visible fat from steak and cut steak into 1-inch pieces. Combine flour, salt and pepper; dredge steak in flour mixture and set aside. Coat a sheet pan with cooking spray. Place meat on pan and coat with spray. Place in a 450° F oven and cook until meat is browned all over. In a large saucepan, mix water with remaining ingredients, stirring well. Add meat, bring to a boil, cover and reduce heat. Simmer for 45 minutes, stirring occasionally. If mixture is not thick enough, thicken with a little cornstarch. Remove bay leaves before serving. Serves 4.

Serve with a 2x2-inch square of cornbread or 1 dinner roll and a spinach salad with tomatoes and lite vinaigrette dressing.
Exchanges: 2 meats, 2½ breads, 2 vegetables, 1½ fats

~~~~~~

Orange Pork Chops

4	4-oz. boneless pork loin chops	⅓	c. reduced-sugar orange
1	bunch green onions, trimmed		marmalade
2	tbsp. Dijon mustard	1	small can mandarin orange
	Vegetable cooking spray		

In a small saucepan mix marmalade and mustard. Stir over medium heat until marmalade is melted. Set aside. Drain oranges and set aside. Place chops on a broiler pan or use outdoor grill. Broil about 4 inches from the heat for about 6 minutes. Turn chops and broil 2 more minutes. Spoon half the glaze over chops. Broil 3 to 4 minutes more or until the chops are no longer pink. Meanwhile slice onions diagonally into 1-inch pieces. Spray a skillet with cooking spray and stir-fry onions 2 minutes until crisp tender. Stir in remaining glaze until heated and add oranges. Serve over chops. Serves 4.

Serve each with ¾ cup potato salad (made with reduced-fat mayonnaise) and 1 cup grilled assorted vegetables.

Exchanges: 3 meats, 2 breads, 1 vegetable, 1 fruit, 1 fat

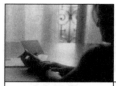

LEADER'S DISCUSSION GUIDE

Life Under
Control

Week One: Life out of Control

1. In this study, group members learned six factors that can cause lives to
    spin out of control. On the board or a sheet of newsprint write the
    numbers 1 through 6 down the left side. Invite different members to
    state the principles from the study. Have one member write each prin-
    ciple on the board or paper.

2. **Before the meeting,** take six index cards and write one of the princi-
    ples on each of the cards and place them in a small paper sack. You
    will lead the group in brainstorming about how each of the factors
    applies to health-related problems. Appoint a timekeeper to monitor
    two-minute intervals for the group discussion. Ask a volunteer to draw
    a card from the sack and read it. Brainstorm the application of that
    factor for two minutes. After two minutes, ask another volunteer to
    draw a second card and read it. Continue this procedure until all six
    principles have been discussed.

3. Ask for volunteers to share which truth they felt was most helpful and
    why. Ask for others to share which truth was most convicting and why.
    Ask for others to share specific changes they want to make as a result
    of the study.

4. Across the top of the board or a large sheet of newsprint, write a scale
    of numbers 1 to 5. Under number 1, write "Discouraged." Under num-
    ber 5, write "Encouraged." Invite group members to form groups of
    three and share their encouragement levels during the past week.
    After all three people have shared, ask group members to pray that
    God will encourage the other two people during the week ahead.

Week Two: Life Under Christ's Control

1. **Before the meeting,** gather a small electric lamp and an extension
    cord (if necessary). Use the lamp to illustrate the Holy Spirit's power
    in our lives. With the lamp unplugged, ask group members to com-

pare the lamp's potential to produce light while unplugged to our potential to live with spiritual power apart from the Holy Spirit's work. Plug in the lamp, turn it on and ask members to share some spiritual principles about our lives and the Spirit's work in us, using the lamp as an illustration. For example: The same way a lamp is designed to draw on power to produce light, so our lives are designed to draw on God's power. Another principle is that if a lamp doesn't produce light, we assume something is wrong; in the same way, if Christians are not experiencing God's power, we assume something is wrong. With the lamp and with our Christian lives, there must be connection with the source of power.

2. Ask for at least two volunteers to share a specific experience in the past week when they sensed the Holy Spirit giving them power. Encourage them to describe how that power influenced their behavior.

3. Have members form groups of three and ask each group to discuss the chart on page 33 that refers to the development of the fruit of the Spirit. Instruct small groups to share two qualities they see developing strongly in their lives and two they don't see now but that they want God to develop. After each person has shared, encourage the other small-group members to affirm the speaker and perhaps even mention other fruit of the Spirit they see in that person's life. After all three people have shared, instruct them to pray for one another, thanking God for developing His fruit in their lives.

4. With the whole group, discuss the warnings in Scripture about limiting the Holy Spirit's work in our lives. On the board or a sheet of newsprint, write "resist," "grieve" and "quench the fire." Ask members to describe ways people limit the Spirit's work as He seeks to give discipline in controlling our habits. How does the Spirit help us control our poor health habits? How can we resist Him, grieve Him or quench His fire?

5. Lead the group in prayer, asking the Holy Spirit to work without limitation in their lives.

Week Three: Thoughts Under Control

1. Ask volunteers to discuss the connection between thoughts and actions. If needed, remind the group that thoughts precede actions; therefore, to control actions we must control our thoughts.

2. Ask a volunteer to recite Philippians 4:8 from memory.

3. Discuss the benefits of having Philippians 4:8 memorized, so they can recite it when our thoughts begin to be negative. Ask two volunteers to describe how they used this verse during the week to help keep their thoughts under control.

4. Explain that the challenge with the type of list contained in Philippians 4:8 is knowing how to use it in our everyday lives. We can affirm that we should think about things that are true, pure, noble, etc., *and* we must think about those words until we understand them and can use them to evaluate our thoughts.

5. **Before the meeting**, gather eight sheets of poster board or newsprint, four felt-tip pens and masking tape. Have members form four groups. Assign two of the words in Philippians 4:8 to each group. Give each group two sheets of poster board or newsprint and a felt-tip pen. Across the top of each sheet, instruct them to write: "I know my thoughts are _____ when . . ." Ask groups to fill in the blank with one of the words from Philippians 4:8 and then complete the sentence. For example: "I know my thoughts are *true* when *they line up with what God has said in the Bible*." After the groups have finished their discussions, ask one member from each group to tape the sheets on the wall and explain what the group discussed. Limit each group's report to one minute.

6. Lead the group in a time of silent prayer. Encourage members to *think* their prayer as an active demonstration that their thoughts can be controlled and used for spiritual purposes.

Week Four: Actions Under Control

1. Begin the meeting by playing a game called Shift the Blame. Have members form a circle. Begin the game by saying to the person on your right "I saw you in the restaurant yesterday eating chocolate cake and ice cream." The person on your right continues the game by saying "Yes, I did, but it was not my fault because . . . ," completing the sentence with some excuse that involves the next person in the circle. For example, the second person could say, "Yes I did, but it was not my fault because it was Dan's birthday and he would have been crushed if I hadn't eaten cake with him." Continue around the circle with each person building on the excuse of the previous person. When the person on your left shifts the blame to you, end the game by saying "I guess it was my fault."

2. Discuss how and why people play Shift the Blame in everyday life.

Then discuss why Christians cannot excuse their behavior and choices by shifting the blame to circumstances or people. Encourage members to draw from the week's study on the power we have as Christians to resist temptation and sin.

4. On the board write the three principles discussed on Day 2, page 55. Explain that one way we can keep our lives under Christ's control is by reminding ourselves of the three principles found in Romans 6:11-13. Sit in a chair in the middle of the circle and tell the group: "I'm at a surprise party, and I'm surrounded by my favorite foods. I don't think I can resist. Give me simple, practical advice based on Romans 6:11-13."

5. Have members review the information about Billy Graham. Invite volunteers to share how Dr. Graham's example of spiritual caution impacted them.

6. Ask volunteers to say a sentence prayer that expresses this idea: "God, because of (state something God has done), I want to (state something you want to do for God)." After several group members have prayed, close the prayer time by asking God to help you and group members to express your gratitude to Him by the way you live.

Week Five: Desires Under Control

1. **Before the meeting,** gather index cards and masking tape. Place a chair in the middle of the room and say that this chair represents a woman named Susan, a person who has developed real contentment in her life. Give each group member an index card and a piece of masking tape. Ask each person to write a sentence describing a specific characteristic we could expect to find in Susan's life because she is a contented person. For example, members could complete this sentence: "I know Susan is content because . . ." Give them a minute or two to complete their cards. Invite them to share what they have written on their cards; then tape the cards to the chair representing Susan.

   After all the cards have been taped to the chair, review the characteristics of contentment that members have written, and add other ideas based on the study. Explain: "We have been assigned the task of helping Susan maintain her contentment. We are concerned that lust, greed and envy may creep into Susan's life; and we want to help her resist them, so we are going to form three task forces to make some recommendations. Each task force will review the material we studied about lust, greed or envy this week. They will summarize the danger and recommend what Susan should do to protect her contentment.

For example, one task force will discuss lust. They will use the material they studied to warn Susan about the ways lust can undermine her contentment. Then they will make several specific recommendations about how Susan can resist the influence of lust in her life. The task forces dealing with greed and envy will follow the same procedure."

Have members form three groups and assign each group one of the three negative influences. Give them six to eight minutes to make their recommendations. Then have each task force appoint a spokesperson who will share the group's recommendations in two minutes or less.

2. Ask for volunteers to pray that God will help the group experience true contentment and resist the negative influences of lust, envy and greed.

Week Six: Self-Esteem Under Control

1. Have the group form pairs and discuss the criteria on which the world bases self-esteem. Allow three minutes; then have several volunteers share their ideas.

2. On the board, draw a vertical line. At the top, write "Inflated self-esteem." At the bottom, write "Inadequate self-esteem." In the middle, write "Healthy self-esteem." Ask group members to think about the people they know and then decide which percentage of the people they know would fall into each group. For example, someone might say "Of the people I know, I guess 25 percent have inflated self-esteem, 50 percent have inadequate self-esteem, and 25 percent have healthy self-esteem." Have volunteers share their estimates. Write the percentages they share. After all have shared, review the percentages group members have assigned to each of the three categories of self-esteem. Discuss: "What patterns do we see in these percentages we have assigned? What could account for the similarities or differences?"

3. Divide the group into two fairly even groups. Tell them they are going to play Point-Counterpoint. Group One will defend the position that inflated self-esteem is the most serious problem they can face. Group Two will take the opposite position. Encourage members to defend assigned positions no matter what they personally believe. Begin the game by allowing one person in Group One to make a brief statement such as "Inflated self-esteem is the most serious problem because . . ." Alternate between Group One and Group Two for five to seven minutes.

4. Ask a volunteer to read Spurgeon's statement on Day 5: "Humility is to make a right estimate of one's self." Discuss: "If a right estimate of one's self can be compared to an accurate map, how do we develop accurate maps of our own lives? How do we view our lives with sober judgment as mentioned in Romans 12:3?"

5. Invite members to share their evaluations of their progress thus far in First Place. Ask them which commitments have been the most difficult to keep. Have them share ways they keep their commitments.

6. Close in prayer, asking volunteers to pray for a healthy self-esteem and to choose a commitment on which to work in the coming week.

Week Seven: Words Under Control

1. Invite someone to read James 1:26. Discuss the impact of our words on our spiritual lives. "How do uncontrolled words render our religion worthless as James states?"

2. Ask members to form groups of three and share which box they checked on Day 2. Have the groups also discuss the challenges they face in listening and remaining silent, rather than talking too much.

3. Have small groups join together to form two large groups. Assign Group One the topic "Words That Stir Up Trouble." Assign Group Two the topic "Words That Hurt People." Have each group review the material they studied and then write three to five examples of their topic and appoint a spokesperson. Give each group two minutes to report to the whole group.

4. Ask volunteers to share what they learned in the Day 5 activity in which they evaluated recent conversations with people in their lives. Have them comment on the degree to which their words helped build their relationships. If they discovered negative patterns in their words, ask them to share changes they plan to make.

5. One reason words are so important is that God uses our words to tell others about His love for them. Share with the group a time when you were talking with another person about Christ and had a special sense that God was using your words to help that person. Ask for others in the group to share similar experiences.

6. Have members turn to Day 5. Words are important because through words we can build our relationship with God. Encourage different people to use each of the five categories of words—worship, praise,

exalt, thank and confess—in their prayers. Close the prayer time by asking God to help members use their words in positive ways.

Week Eight: Spiritual Disciplines Help

1. Begin the meeting by reading Luke 9:23. Have the members form pairs and discuss their answers to this question: "What are you doing in your life right now that indicates you have made any or all of these basic commitments?" Allow five minutes for discussion.

2. In the large group ask for volunteers to share how they completed the exercise on Day 1. Share ideas about how we can deny ourselves; then focus on how to take up our cross; then discuss how to follow Jesus. Keep the discussion focused on practical ways we can express these commitments in our daily lives.

3. One discipline that helps us deny ourselves and self-centered living is a daily quiet time. Share how you have developed this discipline and what it has meant in your spiritual life. Have members review what they wrote on Day 2 about the discipline of a daily quiet time. Ask volunteers to share what they wrote. Focus on practical issues such as when and where they have their quiet times, how they maintain that discipline and what benefits they have experienced.

4. Hand out blank sheets of paper. Ask members to copy the material that you draw on the board or a sheet of newsprint. Draw a large cross (or you could have one already drawn). Where the lines inter-sect, draw a circle and write "Abide in Christ." Ask someone to read John 15:5. At the bottom of the vertical bar, write "Living in the Word." Ask someone to read John 8:31-32. At the top of the vertical bar, write "Praying in faith." Ask someone to read John 15:7. On the right horizontal bar write "Witnessing to the world." Ask someone to read John 15:8 and Acts 1:8. Then explain: "In the same way that we need a balanced diet physically, we need a balanced diet spiritually. The disciplines listed on this cross provide a good guideline to follow."

5. Close in prayer, asking God to help group members build these spiri-tual disciplines in their lives.

Week Nine: Friends Can Help

1. Form groups of three and have members discuss encouragement. Give each group a sheet of paper. Have them fold the paper in half

and write "Encouragement" across the top half of the paper and "Discouragement" on the bottom half. Have each group discuss and complete the following statements: (1) "When I am encouraged, I . . ."; and (2) "When I am discouraged, I . . ." Give each group five minutes to discuss and write their statements. Ask them to share their statements with the whole group.

2. Ask volunteers to share how the group sessions and the members of First Place have encouraged them. Affirm the importance of encouraging one another.

3. Refer to the Day 4 study about blind spots. Share a personal example of a time when involvement with a small group or a friend helped you see a blind spot in your own life. Tell the group how you felt and how you responded. Ask one or two others to share a similar experience. Affirm the role of the First Place group in helping others deal with things in their lives that they might otherwise ignore or miss.

4. Refer to Day 4. Discuss positive ways we can support one another. Help the group focus on the need to carefully consider individuals' needs and backgrounds, so they can be sure their attempts to help have a positive impact.

5. One of the key ways we help one another is by praying for each other. We should follow Paul's example by asking others to pray for us. Give the group an opportunity to ask for prayer for specific needs in their own lives. Close the session in prayer.

Week Ten: A Big Goal and Life Control

1. Discuss why it is important for members to place their weight-loss goals within the broader context of the goals for their whole lives. Help them understand that the spiritual goals for their lives support their health improvement and weight-loss goals. If they want to enjoy better health so that they can serve Christ more fully and glorify Him, then their motivation for success will increase.

2. Our goal is to allow past failures or obstacles as well as successes to provide positive motivation for daily living. Discuss the ways Paul's past was used by God in a positive way in his ministry. How did Paul use the circumstances in his life to live more effectively for Jesus Christ?

3. Invite group members to close their eyes and picture themselves standing before God. What would God say to them? How would He

evaluate their lives? Give the group a minute or two to form this mental picture. Paul wanted to hear God say "Well done, faithful servant." Ask members how they think that desire impacted the way Paul lived. Ask volunteers to share how the desire to hear God say "Well done, faithful servant" impacts the way they live. If no one in the group shares, give your personal testimony of your desire to please God with your life.

4. Refer to the list of obstacles faced by Paul (p. 139). Ask for the group's reaction to the obstacles Paul faced and endured. Invite volunteers to share how Paul's experience makes them feel about the types of obstacles and pressures they face in life. Help them see that just as God helped Paul persevere in the face of incredible challenges, He can help them reach their goals.

5. Form groups of three and share how the commitments to First Place can help them live for Him. Invite them to pray for each other for strength to overcome obstacles and keep their commitments.

PERSONAL WEIGHT RECORD

Week	Weight	+ or -	Goal This Session	Pounds to Goal
1				
2				
3				
4				
5				
6				
7				
8				
9				
10				
11				
12				
13				
Final				

Beginning Measurements

Waist_____ Hips_____ Thighs_____ Chest_____

Ending Measurements

Waist_____ Hips_____ Thighs_____ Chest_____

COMMITMENT RECORDS

How to Fill Out a Commitment Record

The Commitment Record (CR) is an aid for you in keeping track of your accomplishments. Begin a new CR on the morning of the day your class meets. This ensures that your CR is complete before your next meeting. Turn in the CR weekly to your leader.

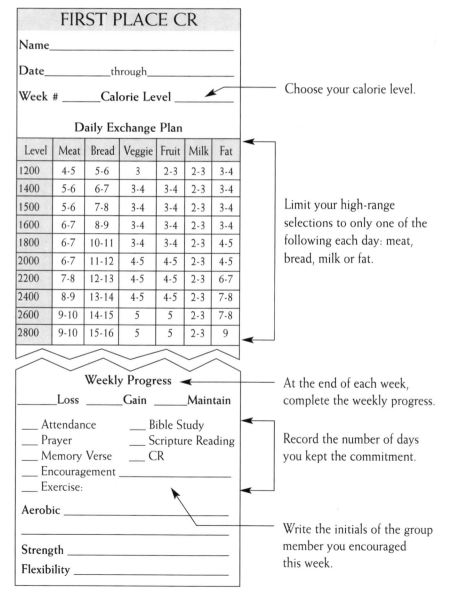

FIRST PLACE CR

Name_____

Date_____through_____

Week # _____Calorie Level _____ — Choose your calorie level.

Daily Exchange Plan

Level	Meat	Bread	Veggie	Fruit	Milk	Fat
1200	4-5	5-6	3	2-3	2-3	3-4
1400	5-6	6-7	3-4	3-4	2-3	3-4
1500	5-6	7-8	3-4	3-4	2-3	3-4
1600	6-7	8-9	3-4	3-4	2-3	3-4
1800	6-7	10-11	3-4	3-4	2-3	4-5
2000	6-7	11-12	4-5	4-5	2-3	4-5
2200	7-8	12-13	4-5	4-5	2-3	6-7
2400	8-9	13-14	4-5	4-5	2-3	7-8
2600	9-10	14-15	5	5	2-3	7-8
2800	9-10	15-16	5	5	2-3	9

Limit your high-range selections to only one of the following each day: meat, bread, milk or fat.

Weekly Progress — At the end of each week, complete the weekly progress.

_____Loss _____Gain _____Maintain

___ Attendance   ___ Bible Study
___ Prayer   ___ Scripture Reading
___ Memory Verse   ___ CR
___ Encouragement _____
___ Exercise:

Aerobic _____

Record the number of days you kept the commitment.

_____

Strength _____

Flexibility _____

Write the initials of the group member you encouraged this week.

DAY 7: Date _____

Morning _____

_____

Midday _____

_____

_____

Evening _____

_____

_____

Snacks _____

_____

_____

___ Meat _____   ☐ Prayer
___ Bread _____   ☐ Bible Study
___ Vegetable _____   ☐ Scripture Reading
___ Fruit _____   ☐ Memory Verse
___ Milk _____   ☐ Encouragement
___ Fat _____   ☐ Water_____

Exercise

Aerobic _____

_____

Strength _____

Flexibility _____

List the foods you have eaten. On this condensed CR it is not necessary to exchange each food choice. It will be the responsibility of each member that the tally marks you list below are accurate regarding each food choice. If you are unsure of an exchange, check the Live-It section of your copy of the *Member's Guide.*

List the daily food exchange choices to the left of the food groups.

Use tally marks for the actual food and water consumed.

Check off commitments completed. Use tally marks to record each 8-oz. serving of water.

List type and duration of exercise.

FIRST PLACE CR

Name _____

Date _____ through _____

Week # _____ Calorie Level _____

Daily Exchange Plan

Level	Meat	Bread	Veggie	Fruit	Milk	Fat
1200	4-5	5-6	3	2-3	2-3	3-4
1400	5-6	6-7	3-4	3-4	2-3	3-4
1500	5-6	7-8	3-4	3-4	2-3	3-4
1600	6-7	8-9	3-4	3-4	2-3	3-4
1800	6-7	10-11	3-4	3-4	2-3	4-5
2000	6-7	11-12	4-5	4-5	2-3	4-5
2200	7-8	12-13	4-5	4-5	2-3	6-7
2400	8-9	13-14	4-5	4-5	2-3	7-8
2600	9-10	14-15	5	5	2-3	7-8
2800	9-10	15-16	5	5	2-3	9

You may always choose the high range of vegetables and fruits. Limit your high range selections to only one of the following: meat, bread, milk or fat.

Weekly Progress

_____ Loss _____ Gain _____ Maintain

_____ Attendance
_____ Prayer
_____ Bible Study
_____ Scripture Reading
_____ Memory Verse
_____ Encouragement:
_____ Exercise
_____ Aerobic
_____ Strength
_____ Flexibility

DAY 5: Date _____

Morning _____

Midday _____

Evening _____

Snacks _____

_____ Meat   ☐ Prayer
_____ Bread   ☐ Bible Study
_____ Vegetable   ☐ Scripture Reading
_____ Fruit   ☐ Memory Verse
_____ Milk   ☐ Encouragement
_____ Fat   Water _____

Exercise
Aerobic _____

Strength _____
Flexibility _____

DAY 6: Date _____

Morning _____

Midday _____

Evening _____

Snacks _____

_____ Meat   ☐ Prayer
_____ Bread   ☐ Bible Study
_____ Vegetable   ☐ Scripture Reading
_____ Fruit   ☐ Memory Verse
_____ Milk   ☐ Encouragement
_____ Fat   Water _____

Exercise
Aerobic _____

Strength _____
Flexibility _____

DAY 7: Date _____

Morning _____

Midday _____

Evening _____

Snacks _____

_____ Meat   ☐ Prayer
_____ Bread   ☐ Bible Study
_____ Vegetable   ☐ Scripture Reading
_____ Fruit   ☐ Memory Verse
_____ Milk   ☐ Encouragement
_____ Fat   Water _____

Exercise
Aerobic _____

Strength _____
Flexibility _____

DAY 1: Date _____

Morning _____
Midday _____
Evening _____
Snacks _____

- ☐ Prayer
- ☐ Bible Study
- ☐ Scripture Reading
- ☐ Memory Verse
- ☐ Encouragement

___ Meat
___ Bread
___ Vegetable
___ Fruit
___ Milk
___ Fat
___ Water

Exercise
Aerobic _____
Strength _____
Flexibility _____

DAY 2: Date _____

Morning _____
Midday _____
Evening _____
Snacks _____

- ☐ Prayer
- ☐ Bible Study
- ☐ Scripture Reading
- ☐ Memory Verse
- ☐ Encouragement

___ Meat
___ Bread
___ Vegetable
___ Fruit
___ Milk
___ Fat
___ Water

Exercise
Aerobic _____
Strength _____
Flexibility _____

DAY 3: Date _____

Morning _____
Midday _____
Evening _____
Snacks _____

- ☐ Prayer
- ☐ Bible Study
- ☐ Scripture Reading
- ☐ Memory Verse
- ☐ Encouragement

___ Meat
___ Bread
___ Vegetable
___ Fruit
___ Milk
___ Fat
___ Water

Exercise
Aerobic _____
Strength _____
Flexibility _____

DAY 4: Date _____

Morning _____
Midday _____
Evening _____
Snacks _____

- ☐ Prayer
- ☐ Bible Study
- ☐ Scripture Reading
- ☐ Memory Verse
- ☐ Encouragement

___ Meat
___ Bread
___ Vegetable
___ Fruit
___ Milk
___ Fat
___ Water

Exercise
Aerobic _____
Strength _____
Flexibility _____

Name _____

Date _____ through _____

Week # _____ Calorie Level _____

Daily Exchange Plan

Level	Meat	Bread	Veggie	Fruit	Milk	Fat
1200	4-5	5-6	3	2-3	2-3	3-4
1400	5-6	6-7	3-4	3-4	2-3	3-4
1500	5-6	7-8	3-4	3-4	2-3	3-4
1600	6-7	8-9	3-4	3-4	2-3	3-4
1800	6-7	10-11	3-4	3-4	2-3	4-5
2000	6-7	11-12	4-5	4-5	2-3	4-5
2200	7-8	12-13	4-5	4-5	2-3	6-7
2400	8-9	13-14	4-5	4-5	2-3	7-8
2600	9-10	14-15	5	5	2-3	7-8
2800	9-10	15-16	5	5	2-3	9

You may always choose the high range of vegetables and fruits. Limit your high range selections to only one of the following: meat, bread, milk or fat.

_____ Loss _____ Gain _____ Maintain

_____ Attendance _____ Bible Study
_____ Prayer _____ Scripture Reading
_____ Memory Verse _____ CR
_____ Encouragement
_____ Exercise
Aerobic _____
Strength _____
Flexibility _____

DAY 5: Date _____

Morning _____

Midday _____

Evening _____

Snacks _____

_____ Meat
_____ Bread
_____ Vegetable
_____ Fruit
_____ Milk
_____ Fat

☐ Prayer
☐ Bible Study
☐ Scripture Reading
☐ Memory Verse
☐ Encouragement
☐ Water _____

Exercise
Aerobic _____

Strength _____
Flexibility _____

DAY 6: Date _____

Morning _____

Midday _____

Evening _____

Snacks _____

_____ Meat
_____ Bread
_____ Vegetable
_____ Fruit
_____ Milk
_____ Fat

☐ Prayer
☐ Bible Study
☐ Scripture Reading
☐ Memory Verse
☐ Encouragement
☐ Water _____

Exercise
Aerobic _____

Strength _____
Flexibility _____

DAY 7: Date _____

Morning _____

Midday _____

Evening _____

Snacks _____

_____ Meat
_____ Bread
_____ Vegetable
_____ Fruit
_____ Milk
_____ Fat

☐ Prayer
☐ Bible Study
☐ Scripture Reading
☐ Memory Verse
☐ Encouragement
☐ Water _____

Exercise
Aerobic _____

Strength _____
Flexibility _____

DAY 1: Date _____

Morning _____

Midday _____

Evening _____

Snacks _____

___ Meat ___	☐ Prayer
___ Bread ___	☐ Bible Study
___ Vegetable ___	☐ Scripture Reading
___ Fruit ___	☐ Memory Verse
___ Milk ___	☐ Encouragement
___ Fat ___	
___ Water ___	

Exercise

Aerobic _____

Strength _____

Flexibility _____

DAY 2: Date _____

Morning _____

Midday _____

Evening _____

Snacks _____

___ Meat ___	☐ Prayer
___ Bread ___	☐ Bible Study
___ Vegetable ___	☐ Scripture Reading
___ Fruit ___	☐ Memory Verse
___ Milk ___	☐ Encouragement
___ Fat ___	
___ Water ___	

Exercise

Aerobic _____

Strength _____

Flexibility _____

DAY 3: Date _____

Morning _____

Midday _____

Evening _____

Snacks _____

___ Meat ___	☐ Prayer
___ Bread ___	☐ Bible Study
___ Vegetable ___	☐ Scripture Reading
___ Fruit ___	☐ Memory Verse
___ Milk ___	☐ Encouragement
___ Fat ___	
___ Water ___	

Exercise

Aerobic _____

Strength _____

Flexibility _____

DAY 4: Date _____

Morning _____

Midday _____

Evening _____

Snacks _____

___ Meat ___	☐ Prayer
___ Bread ___	☐ Bible Study
___ Vegetable ___	☐ Scripture Reading
___ Fruit ___	☐ Memory Verse
___ Milk ___	☐ Encouragement
___ Fat ___	
___ Water ___	

Exercise

Aerobic _____

Strength _____

Flexibility _____

FIRST PLACE CR

Name _____

Date _____ through _____

Week # _____ Calorie Level _____

Daily Exchange Plan

Level	Meat	Bread	Veggie	Fruit	Milk	Fat
1200	4-5	5-6	3	2-3	2-3	3-4
1400	5-6	6-7	3-4	3-4	2-3	3-4
1500	5-6	7-8	3-4	3-4	2-3	3-4
1600	6-7	8-9	3-4	3-4	2-3	3-4
1800	6-7	10-11	3-4	3-4	2-3	4-5
2000	6-7	11-12	4-5	4-5	2-3	4-5
2200	7-8	12-13	4-5	4-5	2-3	6-7
2400	8-9	13-14	4-5	4-5	2-3	7-8
2600	9-10	14-15	5	5	2-3	7-8
2800	9-10	15-16	5	5	2-3	9

You may always choose the high range of vegetables and fruits. Limit your high range selections to only one of the following: meat, bread, milk or fat.

_____ Loss _____ Gain _____ Maintain

_____ Attendance _____ Bible Study
_____ Prayer _____ Scripture Reading
_____ Memory Verse _____ CR
_____ Encouragement
_____ Exercise
Aerobic _____
Strength _____
Flexibility _____

DAY 5: Date _____

Morning _____

Midday _____

Evening _____

Snacks _____

_____ Meat   ☐ Prayer
_____ Bread   ☐ Bible Study
_____ Vegetable ☐ Scripture Reading
_____ Fruit   ☐ Memory Verse
_____ Milk   ☐ Encouragement
_____ Fat   _____ Water

Exercise
Aerobic _____

Strength _____
Flexibility _____

DAY 6: Date _____

Morning _____

Midday _____

Evening _____

Snacks _____

_____ Meat   ☐ Prayer
_____ Bread   ☐ Bible Study
_____ Vegetable ☐ Scripture Reading
_____ Fruit   ☐ Memory Verse
_____ Milk   ☐ Encouragement
_____ Fat   _____ Water

Exercise
Aerobic _____

Strength _____
Flexibility _____

DAY 7: Date _____

Morning _____

Midday _____

Evening _____

Snacks _____

_____ Meat   ☐ Prayer
_____ Bread   ☐ Bible Study
_____ Vegetable ☐ Scripture Reading
_____ Fruit   ☐ Memory Verse
_____ Milk   ☐ Encouragement
_____ Fat   _____ Water

Exercise
Aerobic _____

Strength _____
Flexibility _____

DAY 1: Date _____

Morning _____

Midday _____

Evening _____

Snacks _____

___ Meat ___	☐ Prayer
___ Bread ___	☐ Bible Study
___ Vegetable ___	☐ Scripture Reading
___ Fruit ___	☐ Memory Verse
___ Milk ___	☐ Encouragement
___ Fat ___ Water ___	

Exercise
Aerobic _____

Strength _____

Flexibility _____

DAY 2: Date _____

Morning _____

Midday _____

Evening _____

Snacks _____

___ Meat ___	☐ Prayer
___ Bread ___	☐ Bible Study
___ Vegetable ___	☐ Scripture Reading
___ Fruit ___	☐ Memory Verse
___ Milk ___	☐ Encouragement
___ Fat ___ Water ___	

Exercise
Aerobic _____

Strength _____

Flexibility _____

DAY 3: Date _____

Morning _____

Midday _____

Evening _____

Snacks _____

___ Meat ___	☐ Prayer
___ Bread ___	☐ Bible Study
___ Vegetable ___	☐ Scripture Reading
___ Fruit ___	☐ Memory Verse
___ Milk ___	☐ Encouragement
___ Fat ___ Water ___	

Exercise
Aerobic _____

Strength _____

Flexibility _____

DAY 4: Date _____

Morning _____

Midday _____

Evening _____

Snacks _____

___ Meat ___	☐ Prayer
___ Bread ___	☐ Bible Study
___ Vegetable ___	☐ Scripture Reading
___ Fruit ___	☐ Memory Verse
___ Milk ___	☐ Encouragement
___ Fat ___ Water ___	

Exercise
Aerobic _____

Strength _____

Flexibility _____

Name _____

Date _____ through _____

Week # _____ Calorie Level _____

Daily Exchange Plan

Level	Meat	Bread	Veggie	Fruit	Milk	Fat
1200	4-5	5-6	3	2-3	2-3	3-4
1400	5-6	6-7	3-4	3-4	2-3	3-4
1500	5-6	7-8	3-4	3-4	2-3	3-4
1600	6-7	8-9	3-4	3-4	2-3	3-4
1800	6-7	10-11	3-4	3-4	2-3	4-5
2000	6-7	11-12	4-5	4-5	2-3	4-5
2200	7-8	12-13	4-5	4-5	2-3	6-7
2400	8-9	13-14	4-5	4-5	2-3	7-8
2600	9-10	14-15	5	5	2-3	7-8
2800	9-10	15-16	5	5	2-3	9

You may always choose the high range of vegetables and fruits. Limit your high range selections to only one of the following: meat, bread, milk or fat.

___ Loss ___ Gain ___ Maintain

___ Attendance ___ Bible Study
___ Prayer ___ Scripture Reading
___ Memory Verse ___ CR
___ Encouragement
___ Exercise
Aerobic _____
Strength _____
Flexibility _____

DAY 7: Date _____

Morning _____

Midday _____

Evening _____

Snacks _____

___ Meat ☐ Prayer
___ Bread ☐ Bible Study
___ Vegetable ☐ Scripture Reading
___ Fruit ☐ Memory Verse
___ Milk ☐ Encouragement
___ Fat ☐ Water

Exercise
Aerobic _____
Strength _____
Flexibility _____

DAY 6: Date _____

Morning _____

Midday _____

Evening _____

Snacks _____

___ Meat ☐ Prayer
___ Bread ☐ Bible Study
___ Vegetable ☐ Scripture Reading
___ Fruit ☐ Memory Verse
___ Milk ☐ Encouragement
___ Fat ☐ Water

Exercise
Aerobic _____
Strength _____
Flexibility _____

DAY 5: Date _____

Morning _____

Midday _____

Evening _____

Snacks _____

___ Meat ☐ Prayer
___ Bread ☐ Bible Study
___ Vegetable ☐ Scripture Reading
___ Fruit ☐ Memory Verse
___ Milk ☐ Encouragement
___ Fat ☐ Water

Exercise
Aerobic _____
Strength _____
Flexibility _____

DAY 1: Date _____

Morning _____

Midday _____

Evening _____

Snacks _____

- ☐ Prayer
- ☐ Bible Study
- ☐ Scripture Reading
- ☐ Memory Verse
- ☐ Encouragement

____ Meat
____ Bread
____ Vegetable
____ Fruit
____ Milk
____ Fat
____ Water

Exercise
Aerobic _____
Strength _____
Flexibility _____

DAY 2: Date _____

Morning _____

Midday _____

Evening _____

Snacks _____

- ☐ Prayer
- ☐ Bible Study
- ☐ Scripture Reading
- ☐ Memory Verse
- ☐ Encouragement

____ Meat
____ Bread
____ Vegetable
____ Fruit
____ Milk
____ Fat
____ Water

Exercise
Aerobic _____
Strength _____
Flexibility _____

DAY 3: Date _____

Morning _____

Midday _____

Evening _____

Snacks _____

- ☐ Prayer
- ☐ Bible Study
- ☐ Scripture Reading
- ☐ Memory Verse
- ☐ Encouragement

____ Meat
____ Bread
____ Vegetable
____ Fruit
____ Milk
____ Fat
____ Water

Exercise
Aerobic _____
Strength _____
Flexibility _____

DAY 4: Date _____

Morning _____

Midday _____

Evening _____

Snacks _____

- ☐ Prayer
- ☐ Bible Study
- ☐ Scripture Reading
- ☐ Memory Verse
- ☐ Encouragement

____ Meat
____ Bread
____ Vegetable
____ Fruit
____ Milk
____ Fat
____ Water

Exercise
Aerobic _____
Strength _____
Flexibility _____

Name _____

Date _____ through _____

Week # _____ Calorie Level _____

Daily Exchange Plan

Level	Meat	Bread	Veggie	Fruit	Milk	Fat
1200	4-5	5-6	3	2-3	2-3	3-4
1400	5-6	6-7	3-4	3-4	2-3	3-4
1500	5-6	7-8	3-4	3-4	2-3	3-4
1600	6-7	8-9	3-4	3-4	2-3	3-4
1800	6-7	10-11	3-4	3-4	2-3	4-5
2000	6-7	11-12	4-5	4-5	2-3	4-5
2200	7-8	12-13	4-5	4-5	2-3	6-7
2400	8-9	13-14	4-5	4-5	2-3	7-8
2600	9-10	14-15	5	5	2-3	7-8
2800	9-10	15-16	5	5	2-3	9

You may always choose the high range of vegetables and fruits. Limit your high range selections to only one of the following: meat, bread, milk or fat.

_____ Loss _____ Gain _____ Maintain

_____ Attendance _____ Bible Study
_____ Prayer _____ Scripture Reading
_____ Memory Verse _____ CR
_____ Encouragement
_____ Exercise
_____ Aerobic

_____ Strength _____
_____ Flexibility _____

DAY 5: Date _____

Morning _____

Midday _____

Evening _____

Snacks _____

_____ Meat
_____ Bread
_____ Vegetable
_____ Fruit
_____ Milk
_____ Fat _____ Water

☐ Prayer
☐ Bible Study
☐ Scripture Reading
☐ Memory Verse
☐ Encouragement

Exercise
Aerobic _____

Strength _____
Flexibility _____

DAY 6: Date _____

Morning _____

Midday _____

Evening _____

Snacks _____

_____ Meat
_____ Bread
_____ Vegetable
_____ Fruit
_____ Milk
_____ Fat _____ Water

☐ Prayer
☐ Bible Study
☐ Scripture Reading
☐ Memory Verse
☐ Encouragement

Exercise
Aerobic _____

Strength _____
Flexibility _____

DAY 7: Date _____

Morning _____

Midday _____

Evening _____

Snacks _____

_____ Meat
_____ Bread
_____ Vegetable
_____ Fruit
_____ Milk
_____ Fat _____ Water

☐ Prayer
☐ Bible Study
☐ Scripture Reading
☐ Memory Verse
☐ Encouragement

Exercise
Aerobic _____

Strength _____
Flexibility _____

DAY 1: Date _____

Morning _____

Midday _____

Evening _____

Snacks _____

___ Meat	☐ Prayer
___ Bread	☐ Bible Study
___ Vegetable	☐ Scripture Reading
___ Fruit	☐ Memory Verse
___ Milk	☐ Encouragement
___ Fat ___ Water	

Exercise
Aerobic _____
Strength _____
Flexibility _____

DAY 2: Date _____

Morning _____

Midday _____

Evening _____

Snacks _____

___ Meat	☐ Prayer
___ Bread	☐ Bible Study
___ Vegetable	☐ Scripture Reading
___ Fruit	☐ Memory Verse
___ Milk	☐ Encouragement
___ Fat ___ Water	

Exercise
Aerobic _____
Strength _____
Flexibility _____

DAY 3: Date _____

Morning _____

Midday _____

Evening _____

Snacks _____

___ Meat	☐ Prayer
___ Bread	☐ Bible Study
___ Vegetable	☐ Scripture Reading
___ Fruit	☐ Memory Verse
___ Milk	☐ Encouragement
___ Fat ___ Water	

Exercise
Aerobic _____
Strength _____
Flexibility _____

DAY 4: Date _____

Morning _____

Midday _____

Evening _____

Snacks _____

___ Meat	☐ Prayer
___ Bread	☐ Bible Study
___ Vegetable	☐ Scripture Reading
___ Fruit	☐ Memory Verse
___ Milk	☐ Encouragement
___ Fat ___ Water	

Exercise
Aerobic _____
Strength _____
Flexibility _____

Name _____

Date _____ through _____

Week # _____ Calorie Level _____

Daily Exchange Plan

Level	Meat	Bread	Veggie	Fruit	Milk	Fat
1200	4-5	5-6	3	2-3	2-3	3-4
1400	5-6	6-7	3-4	3-4	2-3	3-4
1500	5-6	7-8	3-4	3-4	2-3	3-4
1600	6-7	8-9	3-4	3-4	2-3	3-4
1800	6-7	10-11	3-4	3-4	2-3	4-5
2000	6-7	11-12	4-5	4-5	2-3	4-5
2200	7-8	12-13	4-5	4-5	2-3	6-7
2400	8-9	13-14	4-5	4-5	2-3	7-8
2600	9-10	14-15	5	5	2-3	7-8
2800	9-10	15-16	5	5	2-3	9

You may always choose the high range of vegetables and fruits. Limit your high range selections to only one of the following: meat, bread, milk or fat.

_____ Loss _____ Gain _____ Maintain

_____ Attendance   _____ Bible Study
_____ Prayer   _____ Scripture Reading
_____ Memory Verse   _____ CR
_____ Encouragement
_____ Exercise
Aerobic _____

Strength _____
Flexibility _____

DAY 7: Date _____

Morning _____
_____

Midday _____
_____

Evening _____
_____

Snacks _____
_____

_____ Meat   ☐ Prayer
_____ Bread   ☐ Bible Study
_____ Vegetable   ☐ Scripture Reading
_____ Fruit   ☐ Memory Verse
_____ Milk   ☐ Encouragement
_____ Fat   Water _____
Exercise
Aerobic _____

Strength _____
Flexibility _____

DAY 6: Date _____

Morning _____
_____

Midday _____
_____

Evening _____
_____

Snacks _____
_____

_____ Meat   ☐ Prayer
_____ Bread   ☐ Bible Study
_____ Vegetable   ☐ Scripture Reading
_____ Fruit   ☐ Memory Verse
_____ Milk   ☐ Encouragement
_____ Fat   Water _____
Exercise
Aerobic _____

Strength _____
Flexibility _____

DAY 5: Date _____

Morning _____
_____

Midday _____
_____

Evening _____
_____

Snacks _____
_____

_____ Meat   ☐ Prayer
_____ Bread   ☐ Bible Study
_____ Vegetable   ☐ Scripture Reading
_____ Fruit   ☐ Memory Verse
_____ Milk   ☐ Encouragement
_____ Fat   Water _____
Exercise
Aerobic _____

Strength _____
Flexibility _____

DAY 1: Date _____

Morning _____

Midday _____

Evening _____

Snacks _____

___ Meat	___ Bread	___ Vegetable	___ Fruit	___ Milk	___ Fat	___ Water

☐ Prayer
☐ Bible Study
☐ Scripture Reading
☐ Memory Verse
☐ Encouragement

Exercise
Aerobic _____
Strength _____
Flexibility _____

DAY 2: Date _____

Morning _____

Midday _____

Evening _____

Snacks _____

___ Meat	___ Bread	___ Vegetable	___ Fruit	___ Milk	___ Fat	___ Water

☐ Prayer
☐ Bible Study
☐ Scripture Reading
☐ Memory Verse
☐ Encouragement

Exercise
Aerobic _____
Strength _____
Flexibility _____

DAY 3: Date _____

Morning _____

Midday _____

Evening _____

Snacks _____

___ Meat	___ Bread	___ Vegetable	___ Fruit	___ Milk	___ Fat	___ Water

☐ Prayer
☐ Bible Study
☐ Scripture Reading
☐ Memory Verse
☐ Encouragement

Exercise
Aerobic _____
Strength _____
Flexibility _____

DAY 4: Date _____

Morning _____

Midday _____

Evening _____

Snacks _____

___ Meat	___ Bread	___ Vegetable	___ Fruit	___ Milk	___ Fat	___ Water

☐ Prayer
☐ Bible Study
☐ Scripture Reading
☐ Memory Verse
☐ Encouragement

Exercise
Aerobic _____
Strength _____
Flexibility _____

FIRST PLACE CR

Name _____

Date _____ through _____

Week # _____ Calorie Level _____

Daily Exchange Plan

Level	Meat	Bread	Veggie	Fruit	Milk	Fat
1200	4-5	5-6	3	2-3	2-3	3-4
1400	5-6	6-7	3-4	3-4	2-3	3-4
1500	5-6	7-8	3-4	3-4	2-3	3-4
1600	6-7	8-9	3-4	3-4	2-3	3-4
1800	6-7	10-11	3-4	3-4	2-3	4-5
2000	6-7	11-12	4-5	4-5	2-3	4-5
2200	7-8	12-13	4-5	4-5	2-3	6-7
2400	8-9	13-14	4-5	4-5	2-3	7-8
2600	9-10	14-15	5	5	2-3	7-8
2800	9-10	15-16	5	5	2-3	9

You may always choose the high range of vegetables and fruits. Limit your high range selections to only one of the following: meat, bread, milk or fat.

_____ Loss _____ Gain _____ Maintain

_____ Attendance _____ Bible Study
_____ Prayer _____ Scripture Reading
_____ Memory Verse _____ CR
_____ Encouragement
_____ Exercise
_____ Aerobic

_____ Strength
_____ Flexibility

DAY 7: Date _____

Morning _____

Midday _____

Evening _____

Snacks _____

_____ Meat   ☐ Prayer
_____ Bread   ☐ Bible Study
_____ Vegetable ☐ Scripture Reading
_____ Fruit   ☐ Memory Verse
_____ Milk   ☐ Encouragement
_____ Fat   _____ Water
Exercise
Aerobic _____

Strength _____
Flexibility _____

DAY 6: Date _____

Morning _____

Midday _____

Evening _____

Snacks _____

_____ Meat   ☐ Prayer
_____ Bread   ☐ Bible Study
_____ Vegetable ☐ Scripture Reading
_____ Fruit   ☐ Memory Verse
_____ Milk   ☐ Encouragement
_____ Fat   _____ Water
Exercise
Aerobic _____

Strength _____
Flexibility _____

DAY 5: Date _____

Morning _____

Midday _____

Evening _____

Snacks _____

_____ Meat   ☐ Prayer
_____ Bread   ☐ Bible Study
_____ Vegetable ☐ Scripture Reading
_____ Fruit   ☐ Memory Verse
_____ Milk   ☐ Encouragement
_____ Fat   _____ Water
Exercise
Aerobic _____

Strength _____
Flexibility _____

DAY 1: Date _____

Morning _____

Midday _____

Evening _____

Snacks _____

- Meat _____ ☐ Prayer
- Bread _____ ☐ Bible Study
- Vegetable _____ ☐ Scripture Reading
- Fruit _____ ☐ Memory Verse
- Milk _____ ☐ Encouragement
- Fat _____ _____ Water _____

Exercise
Aerobic _____
Strength _____
Flexibility _____

DAY 2: Date _____

Morning _____

Midday _____

Evening _____

Snacks _____

- Meat _____ ☐ Prayer
- Bread _____ ☐ Bible Study
- Vegetable _____ ☐ Scripture Reading
- Fruit _____ ☐ Memory Verse
- Milk _____ ☐ Encouragement
- Fat _____ _____ Water _____

Exercise
Aerobic _____
Strength _____
Flexibility _____

DAY 3: Date _____

Morning _____

Midday _____

Evening _____

Snacks _____

- Meat _____ ☐ Prayer
- Bread _____ ☐ Bible Study
- Vegetable _____ ☐ Scripture Reading
- Fruit _____ ☐ Memory Verse
- Milk _____ ☐ Encouragement
- Fat _____ _____ Water _____

Exercise
Aerobic _____
Strength _____
Flexibility _____

DAY 4: Date _____

Morning _____

Midday _____

Evening _____

Snacks _____

- Meat _____ ☐ Prayer
- Bread _____ ☐ Bible Study
- Vegetable _____ ☐ Scripture Reading
- Fruit _____ ☐ Memory Verse
- Milk _____ ☐ Encouragement
- Fat _____ _____ Water _____

Exercise
Aerobic _____
Strength _____
Flexibility _____

FIRST PLACE CR

Name _____

Date _____ through _____

Week # _____ Calorie Level _____

Daily Exchange Plan

Level	Meat	Bread	Veggie	Fruit	Milk	Fat
1200	4-5	5-6	3	2-3	2-3	3-4
1400	5-6	6-7	3-4	3-4	2-3	3-4
1500	5-6	7-8	3-4	3-4	2-3	3-4
1600	6-7	8-9	3-4	3-4	2-3	3-4
1800	6-7	10-11	3-4	3-4	2-3	4-5
2000	6-7	11-12	4-5	4-5	2-3	4-5
2200	7-8	12-13	4-5	4-5	2-3	6-7
2400	8-9	13-14	4-5	4-5	2-3	7-8
2600	9-10	14-15	5	5	2-3	7-8
2800	9-10	15-16	5	5	2-3	9

You may always choose the high range of vegetables and fruits. Limit your high range selections to only one of the following: meat, bread, milk or fat.

_____ Loss _____ Gain _____ Maintain

_____ Attendance _____ Bible Study
_____ Prayer _____ Scripture Reading
_____ Memory Verse _____ CR
_____ Encouragement
_____ Exercise
Aerobic

Strength
Flexibility

DAY 5: Date _____

Morning _____

Midday _____

Evening _____

Snacks _____

_____ Meat ☐ Prayer
_____ Bread ☐ Bible Study
_____ Vegetable ☐ Scripture Reading
_____ Fruit ☐ Memory Verse
_____ Milk ☐ Encouragement
_____ Fat _____ Water

Exercise
Aerobic _____

Strength _____
Flexibility _____

DAY 6: Date _____

Morning _____

Midday _____

Evening _____

Snacks _____

_____ Meat ☐ Prayer
_____ Bread ☐ Bible Study
_____ Vegetable ☐ Scripture Reading
_____ Fruit ☐ Memory Verse
_____ Milk ☐ Encouragement
_____ Fat _____ Water

Exercise
Aerobic _____

Strength _____
Flexibility _____

DAY 7: Date _____

Morning _____

Midday _____

Evening _____

Snacks _____

_____ Meat ☐ Prayer
_____ Bread ☐ Bible Study
_____ Vegetable ☐ Scripture Reading
_____ Fruit ☐ Memory Verse
_____ Milk ☐ Encouragement
_____ Fat _____ Water

Exercise
Aerobic _____

Strength _____
Flexibility _____

DAY 1: Date_____   DAY 2: Date_____   DAY 3: Date_____   DAY 4: Date_____

Morning_____

Midday_____

Evening_____

Snacks_____

_____ Meat   ☐ Prayer
_____ Bread   ☐ Bible Study
_____ Vegetable   ☐ Scripture Reading
_____ Fruit   ☐ Memory Verse
_____ Milk   ☐ Encouragement
_____ Fat   _____ Water

Exercise
Aerobic_____
Strength_____
Flexibility_____

(Day 2, Day 3, and Day 4 repeat the same layout: Morning, Midday, Evening, Snacks; Meat, Bread, Vegetable, Fruit, Milk, Fat; ☐ Prayer, ☐ Bible Study, ☐ Scripture Reading, ☐ Memory Verse, ☐ Encouragement, Water; Exercise — Aerobic, Strength, Flexibility.)

FIRST PLACE CR

Name _____

Date _____ through _____

Week # _____ Calorie Level _____

Daily Exchange Plan

Level	Meat	Bread	Veggie	Fruit	Milk	Fat
1200	4-5	5-6	3	2-3	2-3	3-4
1400	5-6	6-7	3-4	3-4	2-3	3-4
1500	5-6	7-8	3-4	3-4	2-3	3-4
1600	6-7	8-9	3-4	3-4	2-3	3-4
1800	6-7	10-11	3-4	3-4	2-3	4-5
2000	6-7	11-12	4-5	4-5	2-3	4-5
2200	7-8	12-13	4-5	4-5	2-3	6-7
2400	8-9	13-14	4-5	4-5	2-3	7-8
2600	9-10	14-15	5	5	2-3	7-8
2800	9-10	15-16	5	5	2-3	9

You may always choose the high range of vegetables and fruits. Limit your high range selections to only one of the following: meat, bread, milk or fat.

_____ Loss _____ Gain _____ Maintain

_____ Attendance _____ Bible Study
_____ Prayer _____ Scripture Reading
_____ Memory Verse _____ CR
_____ Encouragement
_____ Exercise
Aerobic

Strength _____
Flexibility _____

DAY 5: Date _____

Morning _____

Midday _____

Evening _____

Snacks _____

_____ Meat   □ Prayer
_____ Bread   □ Bible Study
_____ Vegetable □ Scripture Reading
_____ Fruit   □ Memory Verse
_____ Milk   □ Encouragement
_____ Fat   □ Water

Exercise
Aerobic _____

Strength _____
Flexibility _____

DAY 6: Date _____

Morning _____

Midday _____

Evening _____

Snacks _____

_____ Meat   □ Prayer
_____ Bread   □ Bible Study
_____ Vegetable □ Scripture Reading
_____ Fruit   □ Memory Verse
_____ Milk   □ Encouragement
_____ Fat   □ Water

Exercise
Aerobic _____

Strength _____
Flexibility _____

DAY 7: Date _____

Morning _____

Midday _____

Evening _____

Snacks _____

_____ Meat   □ Prayer
_____ Bread   □ Bible Study
_____ Vegetable □ Scripture Reading
_____ Fruit   □ Memory Verse
_____ Milk   □ Encouragement
_____ Fat   □ Water

Exercise
Aerobic _____

Strength _____
Flexibility _____

DAY 1: Date _____

Morning _____

Midday _____

Evening _____

Snacks _____

- ☐ Prayer
- ☐ Bible Study
- ☐ Scripture Reading
- ☐ Memory Verse
- ☐ Encouragement

___ Meat
___ Bread
___ Vegetable
___ Fruit
___ Milk
___ Fat
___ Water

Exercise
Aerobic _____
Strength _____
Flexibility _____

DAY 2: Date _____

Morning _____

Midday _____

Evening _____

Snacks _____

- ☐ Prayer
- ☐ Bible Study
- ☐ Scripture Reading
- ☐ Memory Verse
- ☐ Encouragement

___ Meat
___ Bread
___ Vegetable
___ Fruit
___ Milk
___ Fat
___ Water

Exercise
Aerobic _____
Strength _____
Flexibility _____

DAY 3: Date _____

Morning _____

Midday _____

Evening _____

Snacks _____

- ☐ Prayer
- ☐ Bible Study
- ☐ Scripture Reading
- ☐ Memory Verse
- ☐ Encouragement

___ Meat
___ Bread
___ Vegetable
___ Fruit
___ Milk
___ Fat
___ Water

Exercise
Aerobic _____
Strength _____
Flexibility _____

DAY 4: Date _____

Morning _____

Midday _____

Evening _____

Snacks _____

- ☐ Prayer
- ☐ Bible Study
- ☐ Scripture Reading
- ☐ Memory Verse
- ☐ Encouragement

___ Meat
___ Bread
___ Vegetable
___ Fruit
___ Milk
___ Fat
___ Water

Exercise
Aerobic _____
Strength _____
Flexibility _____

FIRST PLACE CR

Name _____

Date _____ through _____

Week # _____ Calorie Level _____

Daily Exchange Plan

Level	Meat	Bread	Veggie	Fruit	Milk	Fat
1200	4-5	5-6	3	2-3	2-3	3-4
1400	5-6	6-7	3-4	3-4	2-3	3-4
1500	5-6	7-8	3-4	3-4	2-3	3-4
1600	6-7	8-9	3-4	3-4	2-3	3-4
1800	6-7	10-11	3-4	3-4	2-3	4-5
2000	6-7	11-12	4-5	4-5	2-3	4-5
2200	7-8	12-13	4-5	4-5	2-3	6-7
2400	8-9	13-14	4-5	4-5	2-3	7-8
2600	9-10	14-15	5	5	2-3	7-8
2800	9-10	15-16	5	5	2-3	9

You may always choose the high range of vegetables and fruits. Limit your high range selections to only one of the following: meat, bread, milk or fat.

_____ Loss _____ Gain _____ Maintain

_____ Attendance _____ Bible Study
_____ Prayer _____ Scripture Reading
_____ Memory Verse _____ CR
_____ Encouragement
_____ Exercise
Aerobic _____

Strength _____
Flexibility _____

DAY 5: Date _____

Morning _____

Midday _____

Evening _____

Snacks _____

_____ Meat ☐ Prayer
_____ Bread ☐ Bible Study
_____ Vegetable ☐ Scripture Reading
_____ Fruit ☐ Memory Verse
_____ Milk ☐ Encouragement
_____ Fat _____ Water

Exercise
Aerobic _____

Strength _____
Flexibility _____

DAY 6: Date _____

Morning _____

Midday _____

Evening _____

Snacks _____

_____ Meat ☐ Prayer
_____ Bread ☐ Bible Study
_____ Vegetable ☐ Scripture Reading
_____ Fruit ☐ Memory Verse
_____ Milk ☐ Encouragement
_____ Fat _____ Water

Exercise
Aerobic _____

Strength _____
Flexibility _____

DAY 7: Date _____

Morning _____

Midday _____

Evening _____

Snacks _____

_____ Meat ☐ Prayer
_____ Bread ☐ Bible Study
_____ Vegetable ☐ Scripture Reading
_____ Fruit ☐ Memory Verse
_____ Milk ☐ Encouragement
_____ Fat _____ Water

Exercise
Aerobic _____

Strength _____
Flexibility _____

DAY 1: Date _____

Morning _____

Midday _____

Evening _____

Snacks _____

- ___ Meat ___
- ___ Bread ___
- ___ Vegetable ___
- ___ Fruit ___
- ___ Milk ___
- ___ Fat ___
- ___ Water ___

- ☐ Prayer
- ☐ Bible Study
- ☐ Scripture Reading
- ☐ Memory Verse
- ☐ Encouragement

Exercise
Aerobic _____
Strength _____
Flexibility _____

DAY 2: Date _____

Morning _____

Midday _____

Evening _____

Snacks _____

- ___ Meat ___
- ___ Bread ___
- ___ Vegetable ___
- ___ Fruit ___
- ___ Milk ___
- ___ Fat ___
- ___ Water ___

- ☐ Prayer
- ☐ Bible Study
- ☐ Scripture Reading
- ☐ Memory Verse
- ☐ Encouragement

Exercise
Aerobic _____
Strength _____
Flexibility _____

DAY 3: Date _____

Morning _____

Midday _____

Evening _____

Snacks _____

- ___ Meat ___
- ___ Bread ___
- ___ Vegetable ___
- ___ Fruit ___
- ___ Milk ___
- ___ Fat ___
- ___ Water ___

- ☐ Prayer
- ☐ Bible Study
- ☐ Scripture Reading
- ☐ Memory Verse
- ☐ Encouragement

Exercise
Aerobic _____
Strength _____
Flexibility _____

DAY 4: Date _____

Morning _____

Midday _____

Evening _____

Snacks _____

- ___ Meat ___
- ___ Bread ___
- ___ Vegetable ___
- ___ Fruit ___
- ___ Milk ___
- ___ Fat ___
- ___ Water ___

- ☐ Prayer
- ☐ Bible Study
- ☐ Scripture Reading
- ☐ Memory Verse
- ☐ Encouragement

Exercise
Aerobic _____
Strength _____
Flexibility _____

FIRST PLACE CR

Name _____

Date _____ through _____

Week # _____ **Calorie Level** _____

Daily Exchange Plan

Level	Meat	Bread	Veggie	Fruit	Milk	Fat
1200	4-5	5-6	3	2-3	2-3	3-4
1400	5-6	6-7	3-4	3-4	2-3	3-4
1500	5-6	7-8	3-4	3-4	2-3	3-4
1600	6-7	8-9	3-4	3-4	2-3	3-4
1800	6-7	10-11	3-4	3-4	2-3	4-5
2000	6-7	11-12	4-5	4-5	2-3	4-5
2200	7-8	12-13	4-5	4-5	2-3	6-7
2400	8-9	13-14	4-5	4-5	2-3	7-8
2600	9-10	14-15	5	5	2-3	7-8
2800	9-10	15-16	5	5	2-3	9

You may always choose the high range of vegetables and fruits. Limit your high range selections to only one of the following: meat, bread, milk or fat.

_____ Loss   _____ Gain   _____ Maintain

_____ Attendance   _____ Bible Study

_____ Prayer   _____ Scripture Reading

_____ Memory Verse   _____ CR

_____ Encouragement

_____ Exercise

_____ Aerobic

_____ Strength

_____ Flexibility

DAY 7: Date _____

Morning _____

Midday _____

Evening _____

Snacks _____

_____ Meat   ☐ Prayer

_____ Bread   ☐ Bible Study

_____ Vegetable   ☐ Scripture Reading

_____ Fruit   ☐ Memory Verse

_____ Milk   ☐ Encouragement

_____ Fat   Water _____

Exercise

Aerobic _____

Strength _____

Flexibility _____

DAY 6: Date _____

Morning _____

Midday _____

Evening _____

Snacks _____

_____ Meat   ☐ Prayer

_____ Bread   ☐ Bible Study

_____ Vegetable   ☐ Scripture Reading

_____ Fruit   ☐ Memory Verse

_____ Milk   ☐ Encouragement

_____ Fat   Water _____

Exercise

Aerobic _____

Strength _____

Flexibility _____

DAY 5: Date _____

Morning _____

Midday _____

Evening _____

Snacks _____

_____ Meat   ☐ Prayer

_____ Bread   ☐ Bible Study

_____ Vegetable   ☐ Scripture Reading

_____ Fruit   ☐ Memory Verse

_____ Milk   ☐ Encouragement

_____ Fat   Water _____

Exercise

Aerobic _____

Strength _____

Flexibility _____

DAY 1: Date _____

Morning _____

Midday _____

Evening _____

Snacks _____

- ___ Meat _____ □ Prayer
- ___ Bread _____ □ Bible Study
- ___ Vegetable _____ □ Scripture Reading
- ___ Fruit _____ □ Memory Verse
- ___ Milk _____ □ Encouragement
- ___ Fat _____ ___ Water _____

Exercise
Aerobic _____
Strength _____
Flexibility _____

DAY 2: Date _____

Morning _____

Midday _____

Evening _____

Snacks _____

- ___ Meat _____ □ Prayer
- ___ Bread _____ □ Bible Study
- ___ Vegetable _____ □ Scripture Reading
- ___ Fruit _____ □ Memory Verse
- ___ Milk _____ □ Encouragement
- ___ Fat _____ ___ Water _____

Exercise
Aerobic _____
Strength _____
Flexibility _____

DAY 3: Date _____

Morning _____

Midday _____

Evening _____

Snacks _____

- ___ Meat _____ □ Prayer
- ___ Bread _____ □ Bible Study
- ___ Vegetable _____ □ Scripture Reading
- ___ Fruit _____ □ Memory Verse
- ___ Milk _____ □ Encouragement
- ___ Fat _____ ___ Water _____

Exercise
Aerobic _____
Strength _____
Flexibility _____

DAY 4: Date _____

Morning _____

Midday _____

Evening _____

Snacks _____

- ___ Meat _____ □ Prayer
- ___ Bread _____ □ Bible Study
- ___ Vegetable _____ □ Scripture Reading
- ___ Fruit _____ □ Memory Verse
- ___ Milk _____ □ Encouragement
- ___ Fat _____ ___ Water _____

Exercise
Aerobic _____
Strength _____
Flexibility _____

FIRST PLACE CR

Name _____

Date _____ through _____

Week # _____ Calorie Level _____

Daily Exchange Plan

Level	Meat	Bread	Veggie	Fruit	Milk	Fat
1200	4-5	5-6	3	2-3	2-3	3-4
1400	5-6	6-7	3-4	3-4	2-3	3-4
1500	5-6	7-8	3-4	3-4	2-3	3-4
1600	6-7	8-9	3-4	3-4	2-3	3-4
1800	6-7	10-11	3-4	3-4	2-3	4-5
2000	6-7	11-12	4-5	4-5	2-3	4-5
2200	7-8	12-13	4-5	4-5	2-3	6-7
2400	8-9	13-14	4-5	4-5	2-3	7-8
2600	9-10	14-15	5	5	2-3	7-8
2800	9-10	15-16	5	5	2-3	9

You may always choose the high range of vegetables and fruits. Limit your high range selections to only one of the following: meat, bread, milk or fat.

_____ Loss _____ Gain _____ Maintain

_____ Attendance _____ Bible Study
_____ Prayer _____ Scripture Reading
_____ Memory Verse _____ CR
_____ Encouragement
_____ Exercise
Aerobic _____

Strength _____
Flexibility _____

DAY 5: Date _____

Morning _____
_____
_____

Midday _____
_____
_____

Evening _____
_____
_____

Snacks _____
_____
_____

_____ Meat   ☐ Prayer
_____ Bread   ☐ Bible Study
_____ Vegetable   ☐ Scripture Reading
_____ Fruit   ☐ Memory Verse
_____ Milk   ☐ Encouragement
_____ Fat   Water _____

Exercise
Aerobic _____

Strength _____
Flexibility _____

DAY 6: Date _____

Morning _____
_____
_____

Midday _____
_____
_____

Evening _____
_____
_____

Snacks _____
_____
_____

_____ Meat   ☐ Prayer
_____ Bread   ☐ Bible Study
_____ Vegetable   ☐ Scripture Reading
_____ Fruit   ☐ Memory Verse
_____ Milk   ☐ Encouragement
_____ Fat   Water _____

Exercise
Aerobic _____

Strength _____
Flexibility _____

DAY 7: Date _____

Morning _____
_____
_____

Midday _____
_____
_____

Evening _____
_____
_____

Snacks _____
_____
_____

_____ Meat   ☐ Prayer
_____ Bread   ☐ Bible Study
_____ Vegetable   ☐ Scripture Reading
_____ Fruit   ☐ Memory Verse
_____ Milk   ☐ Encouragement
_____ Fat   Water _____

Exercise
Aerobic _____

Strength _____
Flexibility _____

DAY 1: Date _____

Morning _____

Midday _____

Evening _____

Snacks _____

___ Meat ___ ☐ Prayer
___ Bread ___ ☐ Bible Study
___ Vegetable ___ ☐ Scripture Reading
___ Fruit ___ ☐ Memory Verse
___ Milk ___ ☐ Encouragement
___ Fat ___
___ Water ___

Exercise
Aerobic _____
Strength _____
Flexibility _____

DAY 2: Date _____

Morning _____

Midday _____

Evening _____

Snacks _____

___ Meat ___ ☐ Prayer
___ Bread ___ ☐ Bible Study
___ Vegetable ___ ☐ Scripture Reading
___ Fruit ___ ☐ Memory Verse
___ Milk ___ ☐ Encouragement
___ Fat ___
___ Water ___

Exercise
Aerobic _____
Strength _____
Flexibility _____

DAY 3: Date _____

Morning _____

Midday _____

Evening _____

Snacks _____

___ Meat ___ ☐ Prayer
___ Bread ___ ☐ Bible Study
___ Vegetable ___ ☐ Scripture Reading
___ Fruit ___ ☐ Memory Verse
___ Milk ___ ☐ Encouragement
___ Fat ___
___ Water ___

Exercise
Aerobic _____
Strength _____
Flexibility _____

DAY 4: Date _____

Morning _____

Midday _____

Evening _____

Snacks _____

___ Meat ___ ☐ Prayer
___ Bread ___ ☐ Bible Study
___ Vegetable ___ ☐ Scripture Reading
___ Fruit ___ ☐ Memory Verse
___ Milk ___ ☐ Encouragement
___ Fat ___
___ Water ___

Exercise
Aerobic _____
Strength _____
Flexibility _____

FIRST PLACE CR

Name _____

Date _____ through _____

Week # _____ **Calorie Level** _____

Daily Exchange Plan

Level	Meat	Bread	Veggie	Fruit	Milk	Fat
1200	4-5	5-6	3	2-3	2-3	3-4
1400	5-6	6-7	3-4	3-4	2-3	3-4
1500	5-6	7-8	3-4	3-4	2-3	3-4
1600	6-7	8-9	3-4	3-4	2-3	3-4
1800	6-7	10-11	3-4	3-4	2-3	4-5
2000	6-7	11-12	4-5	4-5	2-3	4-5
2200	7-8	12-13	4-5	4-5	2-3	6-7
2400	8-9	13-14	4-5	4-5	2-3	7-8
2600	9-10	14-15	5	5	2-3	7-8
2800	9-10	15-16	5	5	2-3	9

You may always choose the high range of vegetables and fruits. Limit your high range selections to only one of the following: meat, bread, milk or fat.

_____ Loss _____ Gain _____ Maintain

_____ Attendance _____ Bible Study
_____ Prayer _____ Scripture Reading
_____ Memory Verse _____ CR
_____ Encouragement
_____ Exercise
_____ Aerobic

_____ Strength
_____ Flexibility

DAY 5: Date _____

Morning _____

Midday _____

Evening _____

Snacks _____

_____ Meat	☐ Prayer
_____ Bread	☐ Bible Study
_____ Vegetable	☐ Scripture Reading
_____ Fruit	☐ Memory Verse
_____ Milk	☐ Encouragement
_____ Fat	_____ Water

Exercise
Aerobic _____

Strength _____
Flexibility _____

DAY 6: Date _____

Morning _____

Midday _____

Evening _____

Snacks _____

_____ Meat	☐ Prayer
_____ Bread	☐ Bible Study
_____ Vegetable	☐ Scripture Reading
_____ Fruit	☐ Memory Verse
_____ Milk	☐ Encouragement
_____ Fat	_____ Water

Exercise
Aerobic _____

Strength _____
Flexibility _____

DAY 7: Date _____

Morning _____

Midday _____

Evening _____

Snacks _____

_____ Meat	☐ Prayer
_____ Bread	☐ Bible Study
_____ Vegetable	☐ Scripture Reading
_____ Fruit	☐ Memory Verse
_____ Milk	☐ Encouragement
_____ Fat	_____ Water

Exercise
Aerobic _____

Strength _____
Flexibility _____

DAY 1: Date _____ DAY 2: Date _____ DAY 3: Date _____ DAY 4: Date _____

DAY 1: Date _____

Morning _____

Midday _____

Evening _____

Snacks _____

_____ Meat _____ ☐ Prayer
_____ Bread _____ ☐ Bible Study
_____ Vegetable _____ ☐ Scripture Reading
_____ Fruit _____ ☐ Memory Verse
_____ Milk _____ ☐ Encouragement
_____ Fat _____ _____ Water

Exercise
Aerobic _____
Strength _____
Flexibility _____

DAY 2: Date _____

Morning _____

Midday _____

Evening _____

Snacks _____

_____ Meat _____ ☐ Prayer
_____ Bread _____ ☐ Bible Study
_____ Vegetable _____ ☐ Scripture Reading
_____ Fruit _____ ☐ Memory Verse
_____ Milk _____ ☐ Encouragement
_____ Fat _____ _____ Water

Exercise
Aerobic _____
Strength _____
Flexibility _____

DAY 3: Date _____

Morning _____

Midday _____

Evening _____

Snacks _____

_____ Meat _____ ☐ Prayer
_____ Bread _____ ☐ Bible Study
_____ Vegetable _____ ☐ Scripture Reading
_____ Fruit _____ ☐ Memory Verse
_____ Milk _____ ☐ Encouragement
_____ Fat _____ _____ Water

Exercise
Aerobic _____
Strength _____
Flexibility _____

DAY 4: Date _____

Morning _____

Midday _____

Evening _____

Snacks _____

_____ Meat _____ ☐ Prayer
_____ Bread _____ ☐ Bible Study
_____ Vegetable _____ ☐ Scripture Reading
_____ Fruit _____ ☐ Memory Verse
_____ Milk _____ ☐ Encouragement
_____ Fat _____ _____ Water

Exercise
Aerobic _____
Strength _____
Flexibility _____

CONTRIBUTORS

Jody Wilkinson, M.D., M.S., the writer of the Wellness Worksheets for this study, is a physician and exercise physiologist at the Cooper Institute in Dallas, Texas. He trained at the University of Texas Health Science Center in San Antonio, Texas, and Baylor University Medical Center in Dallas. Dr. Wilkinson conducts research on physical activity, nutrition and weight management and has worked with the American Heart Association to develop a health program. He believes strongly in using biblical teaching to motivate people to take care of their physical bodies and enjoy abundant living. Jody and his wife, Natalie, have been married 10 years and have two daughters, Jordan and Sarah, and twin sons, Joel and Cooper.

Scott Wilson, C.E.C., A.A.C., the author of the menu plans in this study, has been cooking professionally for 23 years. A certified executive chef with the American Culinary Federation, he currently works in the Greater Atlanta area as a personal chef and food consultant. Along with serving as the national food consultant for First Place, he is a part-time nutrition teacher at Life University and chef/host of a cable cooking show in the Atlanta area, "Cooking 4 Life." Scott has also authored two cookbooks, *Dining Under the Magnolia* and *Healthy Home Cooking*. In his spare time, he is active in church work and spends time with his wife, Jennifer, and their daughter, Katie.

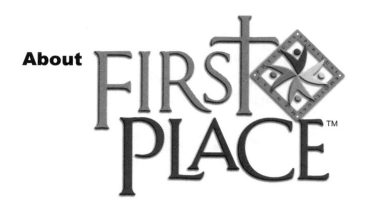

First Place was founded under the providence of God and with the conviction that there is a need for a program which will train the minds, develop the moral character and enrich the spiritual lives of all those who may come within the sphere of its influence.

First Place is dedicated to providing quality information for development of a physical, emotional and spiritual environment leading to a life that honors God in Jesus Christ. As a health-oriented program, First Place will stress the highest excellence and proficiency in instruction with a goal of developing within each participant mastery of all the basics of a lasting healthy lifestyle, so that all may achieve their highest potential in body, mind and spirit. The spiritual development of each participant shall be given high priority so that each may come to the knowledge of Jesus Christ and God's plan and purpose for each life.

First Place offers instruction, encouragement and support to help members experience a more abundant life. Please contact the First Place national office in Houston, Texas at (800) 727-5223 for information on the following resources:

- ❖ Training Opportunities
- ❖ Conferences/Rallies
- ❖ Workshops
- ❖ Fitness Weeks

Send personal testimonies to:

First Place
7401 Katy Freeway
Houston, TX 77024

Join the First Place community at **www.firstplace.org**

THE BIBLE'S WAY TO WEIGHT LOSS

First Place—the Bible-Based Weight-Loss Program
Used Successfully by over a Half Million People!

Are you one of the millions of disheartened dieters who've tried one fad diet after another without success? If so, your search for a successful diet is over! First Place is the proven weight-loss program, born over 20 years ago in the First Baptist Church of Houston.

But First Place does much more than help you take off weight and keep it off. This Bible-based program will transform your life in every way—physically, mentally, spiritually and emotionally. Now's the time to join!

ESSENTIAL FIRST PLACE PROGRAM MATERIALS

Group Leaders need:	Group Members need:

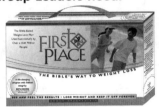

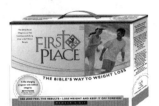

• Group Starter Kit
ISBN 08307.28708

This kit has everything group leaders need to help others change their lives forever by giving Christ first place!

Kit includes:

- *Leader's Guide*
- *Member's Guide*
- *Giving Christ First Place Bible Study* with Scripture Memory Music CD
- *Choosing to Change* by Carole Lewis
- *First Place* by Carole Lewis with Terry Whalin
- *Orientation* Video
- *Nine Commitments* Video
- *Food Exchange Plan* Video

• Member's Kit
ISBN 08307.28694

All the material is easy to understand and spells out principles members can easily apply in their daily lives.

Kit includes:

- *Member's Guide*
- *Choosing to Change* by Carole Lewis
- 13 Commitment Records
- Four Motivational Audiocassettes
- *Prayer Journal*
- Scripture Memory Verses: *Walking in the Word*

• First Place Bible Study

Giving Christ First Place Bible Study with Scripture Memory Music CD

Bible Study
ISBN 08307.28643

Other Bible studies available

Available at your local Christian bookstore or by calling 1-800-4-GOSPEL.
Join the First Place community at **www.firstplace.org**

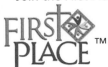

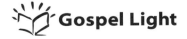

11063

Bible Studies
to Help You Put Christ
First

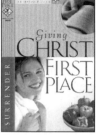

Giving Christ First Place
Bible Study
ISBN 08307.28643
Now Available

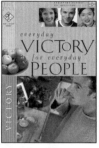

**Everyday Victory
for Everyday People**
Bible Study
ISBN 08307.28651
Now Available

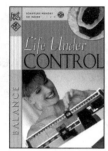

Life Under Control
Bible Study
ISBN 08307.29305
Now Available

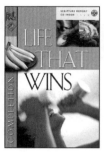

Life That Wins
Bible Study
ISBN 08307.29240
Now Available

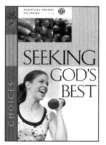

Seeking God's Best
Bible Study
ISBN 08307.29259
Available April 2002

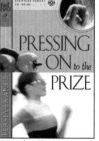

Pressing On to the Prize
Bible Study
ISBN 08307.29267
Available April 2002

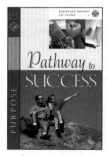

Pathway to Success
Bible Study
ISBN 08307.29275
Available July 2002

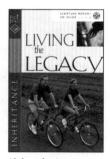

Living the Legacy
Bible Study
ISBN 08307.29283
Available July 2002

Available at your local Christian bookstore or by
calling 1-800-4-GOSPEL.

Join the First Place community at **www.firstplace.org** 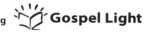 **Gospel Light**

11062

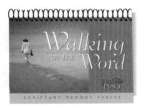
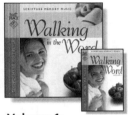
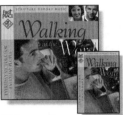
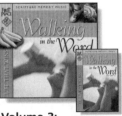
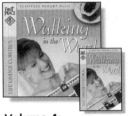
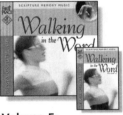
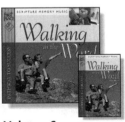
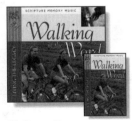
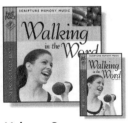

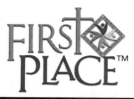

Available from your Gospel Light supplier

First Place Resource Order Form

TITLE	ISBN/SPCN	QTY	PRICE	ITEM TOTAL
First Place Group Starter Kit ($198 Value!)	08307.28708		149.99	
First Place Member's Kit ($101 Value!)	08307.28694		79.99	
First Place (Lewis/Whalin) (included in Group Starter Kit)	08307.28635		18.99	
Choosing to Change (Lewis) (included in Member's and Group Starter Kits)	08307.28627		8.99	
Giving Christ First Place Bible Study w/Scripture Memory Music CD (included in Group Starter Kit)	08307.28643		19.99	
Everyday Victory for Everyday People Bible Study w/Scripture Memory Music CD	08307.28651		19.99	
Life That Wins Bible Study w/ Scripture Memory Music CD	08307.29240		19.99	
Life Under Control Bible Study w/ Scripture Memory Music CD	08307.29305		19.99	
Pressing On to the Prize Bible Study w/ Scripture Memory Music CD	08307.29267		19.99	
Seeking God's Best Bible Study w/ Scripture Memory Music CD	08307.29259		19.99	
Living the Legacy Bible Study w/ Scripture Memory Music CD	08307.29283		19.99	
Pathway to Success Bible Study w/ Scripture Memory Music CD	08307.29275		19.99	
Prayer Journal (included in Member's Kit)	08307.29003		9.99	
Motivational Audiocassettes (pkg. of 4) (included in Member's Kit)	607135.005988		29.99	
Commitment Records (pkg. o f 13) (included in Member's Kit)	08307.29011		6.99	
Scripture Memory Verses: Walking in the Word (included in Member's Kit)	08307.28996		14.99	
Leader's Guide (included in Group Starter Kit)	08307.28678		19.99	
Food Exchange Plan Video (included in Group Starter Kit)	607135.006138		29.99	
Orientation Video (included in Group Starter Kit)	607135.005940		29.99	
Nine Commitments Video (included in Group Starter Kit)	607135.005957		39.99	
Giving Christ First Place Scripture Memory Music CD	607135.005902		9.99	
Giving Christ First Place Scripture Memory Music Cassette	607135.005919		6.99	
Everyday Victory for Everyday People Scripture Memory Music CD	607135.005926		9.99	
Everyday Victory for Everyday People Scripture Memory Music Cassette	607135.005933		6.99	
Life Under Control Scripture Memory Music CD	607135.006213		9.99	
Life Under Control Scripture Memory Music Cassette	607135.006206		6.99	
Life That Wins Scripture Memory Music CD	607135.006237		9.99	
Life That Wins Scripture Memory Music Cassette	607135.006220		6.99	
Seeking God's Best Scripture Memory Music CD	607135.006244		9.99	
Seeking God's Best Scripture Memory Music Cassette	607135.006251		6.99	
Pressing On to the Prize Scripture Memory Music CD	607135.006268		9.99	
Pressing On to the Prize Scripture Memory Music Cassette	607135.006275		6.99	
Pathway to Success Scripture Memory Music CD	607135.006282		9.99	
Pathway to Success Scripture Memory Music Cassette	607135.006299		6.99	
Living the Legacy Scripture Memory Music CD	607135.006305		9.99	
Living the Legacy Scripture Memory Music Cassette	607135.006312		6.99	

PRICES SUBJECT TO CHANGE.

11052

Total : $_____